DATE DUE

Epidemiologic Methods
for Health Policy

Epidemiologic Methods for Health Policy

ROBERT A. SPASOFF

New York   Oxford
OXFORD UNIVERSITY PRESS
1999

Oxford University Press

Oxford   New York
Athens   Auckland   Bangkok   Bogotá   Buenos Aires   Calcutta
Cape Town   Chennai   Dar es Salaam   Delhi   Florence   Hong Kong   Istanbul
Karachi   Kuala Lumpur   Madrid   Melbourne   Mexico City   Mumbai
Nairobi   Paris   São Paulo   Singapore   Taipei   Tokyo   Toronto   Warsaw

and associated companies in
Berlin   Ibadan

Copyright © 1999 by Oxford University Press, Inc.

Published by Oxford University Press, Inc.
198 Madison Avenue, New York, New York 10016

Oxford is a registered trademark of Oxford University Press

Library of Congress Cataloging-in-Publication Data
Spasoff, R. A.
Epidemiologic methods for health policy /
Robert A. Spasoff.
p. cm.   Includes bibliographical references and index.
ISBN 0-19-511499-X
1. Epidemiology.   2. Medical policy.
I. Title.
RA652.S67   1999   362.1—dc21   98-50116

9 8 7 6 5 4 3 2 1

Printed in the United States of America
on acid-free paper

Preface

Why another book on epidemiology and health policy? Because as the study of the health of populations, epidemiology can make a unique contribution to health policy, and because no book focusing on the most relevant methods appears to exist at present. Textbooks of general epidemiology tend to ignore this subject and the descriptive epidemiologic methods that are most relevant to it, and to focus almost entirely on etiological research. Several books on epidemiology and health policy have dealt more with examples than with methods, and have aimed at very wide audiences, including both epidemiologists and policymakers; none appears to be in print now.

This text is intended for persons who have completed a basic course in epidemiology, especially graduate students and epidemiologists who wish to apply their discipline to the development and evaluation of health policy. I use it as the textbook for a course in epidemiology and health policy. Many readers will work in government, health planning councils, public health units, or policy institutes, although some may work in professional organizations or industry. Others will work in universities, but want their work to be directly relevant to the above organizations. The book is intended as a contribution to the development of evidence-based policymaking. It is not an introduction to epidemiology for policymakers, although it attempts to introduce policy to epidemiologists. Since there is usually more than one way to look at policy, two or more authorities are quoted in many cases, to give the reader a sense of the range of approaches available.

The book is concerned mainly with *public* policy, the policies of governments, and is oriented toward developed countries. A major decision in producing such a book concerns the distinction between policy and programs, specifically whether to address health services planning and evaluation at the program level. This book does not address the planning and evaluation of specific programs, although it does cover the assessment of concepts or approaches that are reflected in specific programs. Thus, the book considers epidemiologic methods that might be used to assess the evidence regarding the community effectiveness of early-discharge programs from hospitals, but not methods to evaluate the early-discharge program in a specific city at a specific time. Similarly, it does not directly address personal health services, although it will be more relevant to public health services, which have more of a policy orientation.

The book has two parts. Part I deals with general issues. Chapter 1 introduces the subject of public policy and its formation, and reviews the potential contribution of epidemiology to it. The chapter then addresses ethical and political issues faced by epidemiologists working in policy and ends with a few comments on communications. Chapter 2 presents selected epidemiologic methods that are relevant to the whole health policy cycle, borrowing heavily from demography and lightly from economics. In recognition of the readers' (possible) and the author's (undoubted) limitations, mathematical content is confined to elementary algebra. Chapter 3 focuses on health data, important raw material for health policy, reviewing their sources and uses and some methods for handling them.

Part II systematically follows the policy cycle, presenting and discussing the epidemiologic methods that are useful at each step, with examples. Chapter 4 addresses measurement of the health of populations, including developing a population health profile, identifying health needs and risks, and assessing the evidence for the causes of health problems (with emphasis on the role of ecological studies). Chapter 5 considers the assessment of evidence on the effectiveness, efficiency, potential coverage, and feasibility of potential interventions available to address health problems, and discusses the contribution of meta-analysis to health policy. Chapter 6 tackles the difficult area of making choices among the available alternatives, beginning with the choice between prevention and treatment, proceeding to the use of disease modeling, and ending with the setting of priorities. Chapter 7 deals with policy implementation, including definition of health goals, allocation of health resources, and ensuring that the necessary data are collected for monitoring and evaluation. Finally, Chapter 8 closes the policy loop by considering the evaluation of policy and the continuing monitoring of health, including the role of surveillance in the identification of emerging problems.

This book grows from more than 25 years of teaching epidemiology and working with persons in governments, public health departments, and health planning councils. I hope that it will help other epidemiologists to stumble less often and make their epidemiologic contributions more efficiently.

March 1999   R.A.S.
Ottawa, Ontario

Acknowledgments

The University of Ottawa granted a sabbatical leave during which the initial hard thinking for this book was conducted, and allowed the writing of a textbook as a legitimate academic activity. Louise Gunning-Schepers provided a wonderfully supportive environment during that year at the Institute of Social Medicine, University of Amsterdam, not least through her inspired demonstrations of the possibilities for applying epidemiology to health policy. A WHO Travel Fellowship permitted additional study of European experience. My colleagues at the University of Ottawa, Nick Birkett, John Last, Andreas Laupacis, Ian McDowell and Rama Nair, allowed me to bounce ideas off them and corrected many misapprehensions. The students in my graduate course on Epidemiology and Health Policy have enjoyed identifying fuzzy thinking and opaque writing. Parts of Chapter 3 are based on a Community Health Research Unit Working Paper, prepared in 1993 with Geoff Dunkley and David Gilkes. Louise Gunning-Schepers and Menno Reijneveld read an earlier draft of the entire book, and provided much useful advice on both content and organization. Doug Angus and Don Wigle read and corrected the first chapter. Jeffrey House at Oxford University Press provided continuing guidance and exhibited great patience, while the comments from the readers retained by the Press improved the book immensely. Beyond that, the usual disclaimers.

Contents

I

CONCEPTS, METHODS, AND DATA

Epidemiologists need to understand the policy process and to possess relevant expertise if they are to work effectively within it. Population health data are essential raw material for the construction of health policy. Epidemiologic methods can help convert health data into health information and ultimately into health intelligence, the basis upon which decisions are (ideally) made.

1

Policy, Public Policy, and Health Policy

How healthy is the population? Is its health becoming better or worse? Are some population groups significantly less healthy than others? What are the main health problems? What are the trends in these problems, and what is the picture likely to be in the future? Should the government do anything about any of these problems? Which ones? What interventions are available? Which ones "work"? Would they work in the population in question? At which segments of the population should they be directed? What would be their overall impact on the health and quality of life of the population? How should the government decide which interventions should be implemented? How will the government know if its new policy is successful?

1.1 What Is Policy?

The above questions call for policy decisions. Traditionally, these matters were left mainly to individual clinicians, but with increasingly complex and expensive care and an empowered population, that approach is no longer tenable. The result is that more and more issues are becoming topics for public policy—in the form of regulations, educational programs, funding, or direct provision of services (of course, public health services have always been public). These issues raise difficult questions, and policymakers are often faced by more advice than evidence, but decisions must be made nonetheless. The thesis of this book is that epidemiology can help to inform these decisions, and its purpose is to provide epidemiologists with the knowledge and skills to fill this role. First, it is necessary for the epidemiologist to know something about policy and its uses.

Policy

For the purpose of this book, *policy* is a set of principles guiding decision making. Walt (1994:42–3) distinguishes between *systemic* (macro) policy, which determines the basic characteristics of a society, and *sectoral* (micro) policy, which concerns lower-level decisions within it. Policy provides a framework against which proposals can be tested and progress measured. Policies are necessary if an organization's actions are to be consistent with one another, or even aimed in the same direction; without them, the organization's actions will be unfocused and fragmented, and the organization is likely to be ineffective. All organizations have policies, although they may not be written. Ideally, a policy contains a definition of the *problem* being addressed, a statement of *goals* (the desired state of affairs), and at least the broad outlines of the *instruments* (approaches and activities) by which the goals are to be achieved (Pal, 1992:11). Policymaking includes implementation, and policy usually cannot be considered to exist until it is actually carried out, a perspective reflected in Walt's definition, "a series of more or less related activities and their intended and unintended consequences for those concerned" (Walt, 1994:41).

Public Policy

Public policy refers to the policies of governments. The U.S. National Library of Medicine's Medical Science Headings define public policy (MeSH #798) as "a course or method of action selected, usually by government, from among alternatives to guide and determine present and future decisions." But policy can also take the form of inaction, as in "a course of action or inaction chosen by public authorities to address a given problem or interrelated set of problems" (Pal, 1992:2). Because these actions or inactions are "chosen," policymaking must involve conscious decisions. Private organizations and even individuals have policies, but this book applies primarily to public policy, as do most publications on policy. The identification of policy with the public sector and its close relationship to the political process is consistent with use of the same word for "policy" and "politics" in many languages .

Health Policy

This book is about *health policy,* which concerns the whole field of health, going well beyond health care to encompass the determinants of health. A recent Dutch policy document (Ruwaard et al., 1994:27) defines its scope: "Health policy in the broadest sense is understood here as the actions of government and other players which are aimed at maintaining and improving the population's state of health. More specifically, a distinction can be made between *health-care policy, prevention policy* and *intersectoral policy.*" This last kind of policy is related to the World Health Organization's (WHO) concept of *healthy public policy* which "puts health on the agenda of policymakers in all sectors and at all levels, directing them to be aware of the health consequences of their decisions and to accept their responsibilities for health" (World Health Organization, 1986). Many of the factors that influence health do not fall within the ambit of a country's Ministry of Health. It can be extremely difficult to achieve the necessary intersectoral cooperation; budgets are fixed by ministry or department, and other ministries do not have health as a priority. The National Library of Medicine defines health policy (MeSH #1845) more narrowly as "decisions, usually developed by government policymakers, for determining present and future objectives pertaining to the health care system." Its subheadings, health care reform and nutrition policy, are nearly as narrow in scope. Health policy is not always public: "Health policy is courses of action that affect the set of institutions, organisations, services and funding arrangements of the care system. It goes beyond health services, however, and includes actions and intended actions by public, private and voluntary organisations that have an impact on health" (Walt, 1994:41).

1.2 Who Makes Policy?

The *policy system* is the overall institutional pattern within which policies are made, comprising policies, stakeholders, and the environment (Dunn, 1981:46). Three patterns have been defined, although these rarely exist in pure form (van der Grinten, 1996:137–8). Although developed to apply to political jurisdictions, the principles are somewhat applicable to organizations like companies and professional associations.

At one extreme is a *unicentric* policy system in which one authority, generally government, is all-powerful, being the only important decision-making entity. The result is a regulated system in which government allocates and coordinates tasks. Examples are totalitarian governments and perhaps some of the Southeast Asian democracies.

At the other extreme is a *multicentric* policy system, essentially a marketplace, in which many autonomous actors compete. Government acts as referee, guardian of minimal standards, and facilitator of desired behavior on the part of the other players, who will only play if a particular policy is to their own benefit (in fact, governments usually find it necessary to engage in fairly extensive regulation to deal with market failures). Rather than controlling the environment, government must adapt its organization to the existing environment. The English-speaking democracies are examples.

The third, intermediate type of policy system is a *pluricentric* system, in which the model is a network. Power is shared by a small number of interdependent actors including government, employers, and labor, who must work together to achieve their various objectives. Policy can be successfully implemented only when there is widespread support among the important players. This "neocorporatist" policy system has been exemplified by Japan and Germany in recent decades.

A country's policy system influences how the participants in policy-making interact, as discussed in Section 1.3. It also determines their relative importance, and thus their importance as targets for the epidemiologist's communications. But first the range of participants must be identified. Countries vary tremendously, so it is not easy to generalize, but democracies have certain features in common. The most important players are politicians, civil servants, advisors, and interest groups.

The *government* (government of the day, or party or parties in power) sets the overall policy direction (macro policy). In parliamentary democracies, this is fairly straightforward, since the legislative and executive functions are combined, although multiparty coalitions complicate the issue. In the United States, both Congress and the President participate in policy formation, though not always amicably. The *prime minister* or president is instrumental in developing macro policy and serves as its main exponent. It is rare for the prime minister or president to be particularly interested in health (exceptions are found in Box 1-1), and other members of the cabinet often see the sector as a bottomless pit into which they throw money.

The *minister of health* is responsible for health policy and is thus the central figure in health policy development, which includes preparing policy, persuading the cabinet and the legislature to accept it, and explaining it to the public. But for several reasons, it is not common for a minister of health to make a lasting impression on policy. In parliamentary systems, ministers almost never have expertise in the health field when they are first appointed to office; indeed, it is sometimes argued that a health professional would be in conflict of interest as minister of health. A new minister of health therefore needs to be educated on health and its determinants. In the United States, the secretary (the equivalent of minister) of Health and Human Services does not need to be an elected representative, so that person is more likely to come to the office with

---

Box 1-1 Some government leaders get involved in health

An example of a government leader taking a very major interest in health was Premier Tommy Douglas's introduction of public health care insurance in the Canadian province of Saskatchewan in 1947 (for hospital coverage) and 1962 (for coverage of physicians' services); the program was later extended to the entire country. But commitment on the part of the leader is not sufficient. Political conditions must be conducive to introduction of a major policy, as they were in the 1960s when the Johnson administration in the U.S. introduced Medicare and Medicaid, but not in the 1990s when the Clinton administration tried to introduce a universal health insurance program. Of course, the major responsibility for health policy in both Canada and the United States lies with the provinces and states.

relevant expertise, gained in the social sector. Ministers must deal with a range of interest groups and short-term crises, which tend to prevent them from thinking about long-range issues. They remain in office at the pleasure of the prime minister or president, and may be removed from office for a variety of reasons, including deficient or excessive competence, as well as electoral defeat. Their tenure is often fairly short. Finally, the minister of health usually has limited influence in the financial sphere, where real political power resides; in some systems, the minister of health is not even a member of the (inner) cabinet. Despite these factors, some ministers provide significant leadership in health policy (Box 1-2).

The influence of individual *members of the legislature* (Parliament, Congress), depends upon the extent to which party discipline is enforced. In some parliamentary systems they have little influence over policy, since their main responsibility (unless they rise to cabinet status) is to vote for the government's bills. U.S. Congressmen (especially senators) have much greater influence because of the important role of Congress in policy development and the committee system that operates there.

Ministers' executive assistants (who go by various titles) are usually young, often bright, and always appointed on the basis of political connections; they rarely possess health expertise. They are responsible only to the minister, and their tenure in office is often short. There is every indication that they play an important role in the development of health policy, through their own direct access and their control over the access of others to the minister. They are therefore important targets for epidemiologic communications.

Civil servants are the only "permanent" players within government, although in some systems the most senior levels change with the government. Such systems permit the appointment of individuals with specialized expertise, although the appointments are also influenced by political considerations. In fully professional systems (where civil servants have career appointments), the senior levels have traditionally risen through the ranks in their own departments, although there is a recent tendency toward senior levels being taken over by professional managers, persons

---

Box 1-2 Ministers can have a big influence

Two Canadian ministers were instrumental in defining health promotion (or encouraging it be defined by their ministries), culminating in the publication of *A New Perspective on the Health of Canadians* in 1974 (the Lalonde Report) and *Achieving Health for All* in 1986 (the Epp Report). Both these documents significantly influenced Canadian health policy, at least in the short term. Also see Box 1-4.

trained in generic management skills. They may be moved into health from unrelated fields and then (about the time that they begin to understand the health field) moved to other ministries. The senior civil servant in the ministry of health (deputy minister of health or assistant secretary for health) shares the central role in policy development with the minster or secretary. The civil service is responsible for most of the process of policy development and implementation, although with the downsizing of governments, some policy development tasks are being contracted out to consultants. Collectively, the civil service often possesses enormous subject expertise, but there are complex relations within it that may prevent this expertise from being optimally used. Policy groups may be far removed (organizationally, psychologically, and physically) from the operating branches, which contain the persons with subject expertise; in some systems these groups may be entirely outside the ministry of health, in a central agency remote from real-world problems. The result of these factors is that those civil servants who possess the subject expertise needed to develop policy may lack the opportunity to do so, and vice versa; the exceptions (Box 1-3) can offer real opportunities. Civil servants may be unwilling to consider policy proposals that they believe will not be supported by the government of the day. In some systems, civil servants are expected to protect the minister from criticism or adverse publicity, a responsibility that conflicts with their role in policy development. In the United States, the surgeon general occupies an influential and somewhat independent position, from which it is possible to have a major impact on health policy. The same can be said for the chief medical officer in the United Kingdom.

Temporary or ad hoc *committees* (task forces) and quasi-permanent *advisory groups and councils* are often appointed by governments to advise on aspects of health policy. Their reports may make an important contribution to policy development, but may also be ignored, unless their recommendations coincide with what the government wants to do (see Box 1-4). Consensus conferences serve a somewhat similar purpose in bringing together experts and interest groups to develop policy recommenda-

---

Box 1-3 Civil servants can drive policy

Civil servants in the Health Promotion Directorate of Health and Welfare Canada provided intellectual leadership to the Canadian health promotion movement throughout the 1970s and 1980s and appeared to provide policy leadership for the whole department. They wrote the two documents mentioned in Box 1-2, and were prominent and credible in academic circles.

Box 1-4. When do advisory commissions work?

Two Canadian provinces provide a contrast. By the time the important Castonguay Commission reported to the Quebec government in the early 1970s, its Chair (who was an accountant by training, but who had developed much health expertise during his chairmanship of the commission) had been elected to the National Assembly and appointed Minister of Health. Again in the early 1990s, an eminent medical specialist in public health, who had recently chaired another important advisory committee to the government, became Minister of Health. Can there be any relationship to the fact that Quebec has consistently led the country in health policy during this period? More typical was the experience in neighboring Ontario, where the government followed the advice of an advisory commission and formed an intersectoral Premier's Council on Health Strategy in 1987. Comprising cabinet ministers and representatives of the health sector and the general public, the Council produced several visionary documents. But the government changed in 1990, and the new government appeared to identify the Council with the previous government (despite the fact that the Council's directions appeared highly consistent with those of the new government). The Council languished, and after several name-changes and a further change in government, it was terminated. All of this points to the importance of building a wide constituency, including all political parties. It also points to more fundamental differences between the two provinces, Quebec being more statist, or somewhat closer to a unicentric pattern and thus more willing to use government intervention, and Ontario being more pluralist, which is pluricentric or even multicentric.

---

tions on a specific issue. The methods for conducting them are well developed, particularly in the United States (McGlynn et al., 1990).

Research institutes. Free-standing policy institutes have become important sources of policy analysis and advice, often providing great expertise. But their credibility is limited by their responsibility to their sponsors (funders), who are most often business interests. University research groups may have greater credibility, but their scope may also be somewhat limited by their dependence upon government or industrial funding.

Interest groups abound in health as in other fields. Three groupings directly relevant to health policy are (1) industry, e.g., manufacturers of drugs and medical devices, insurance companies, and hospital companies, which are becoming increasingly powerful; (2) professional organizations of hospitals, doctors, nurses, and public health professionals, which are less powerful than the previous category; and (3) consumer groups, e.g., patients' associations, which are even less powerful. The first two categories in particular establish well-funded lobbies adjacent to government, develop lasting relationships with politicians and civil servants, and have considerable policy expertise—sometimes more than exists in government. They are therefore in a position to have great influence, and in some cases responsibility for certain programs is delegated to them; e.g., the Canadian government delegated responsibility for national AIDS education to the Canadian Public Health Association, and for maintaining a physician database to the Canadian Medical Association. In neocorporatist structures like those in Germany or The Netherlands, private groups take on some of the usual functions of government, such as administration of universal health insurance. Even more important than the health-related groups are business groups, e.g., multinational corporations and chambers of commerce, which currently dictate the overall policy directions of governments and thus determine the scope for health policy development. In principle, labor unions or religious groups could do the same.

The *general public* has relatively limited opportunity to influence health policy in most countries, beyond going to the polls to vote every few years, but they may be given a more important role through the recent move toward recall provisions and referenda in North America. Public opinion polls inform the government of at least the broad priorities of the public, and some members of the public participate in political parties or other organizations having policy interests.

1.3 How Is Policy Made?

Discussions of the policymaking process tend to identify three broad models ("theories") loosely corresponding to the policy systems described in the previous section. Although the categories defined by different authors are not identical, the two extreme forms are reasonably consistent.

The first model is *rational theory* (van der Grinten, 1996:138), also called *rational-comprehensive* (Dunn, 1981:226) or *rational-deductive* theory (Walt, 1994:46). This top-down approach is characterized by formal planning, with objectives and targets. The theory assumes consensus among stakeholders, adequate knowledge to support policymaking, and a stable environment in which the one important actor (generally the government) can apply the plan sequentially. The term *synoptic* is sometimes used for situations in which there is more limited knowledge and room for maneuver (Walt, 1994:46). The conditions for this model are most likely to be found in a unicentric policy system, e.g., the five-year plans of the former Eastern Bloc, and of many developing countries. In this mode policy matters, and epidemiology could play a big role in informing the grand plans. But the conditions necessary for this model rarely obtain, and even when they do, the approach has not been particularly successful (consider the Eastern Bloc). Lindblom (1959) has argued that it cannot work, because the human mind is unable to deal with the complexity of policy problems. Furthermore, Arrow's (1970:59–60) "possibility theorem" shows that it is impossible for decision makers in a democratic society to meet the conditions of the rational theory, because individual preferences cannot be aggregated to produce a single solution that is best for all parties. A basic problem is that there is not one rationality but many rationalities, with different perspectives.

The second model is *disjointed incrementalism* (Braybrooke and Lindblom, 1963: 82), also called *muddling through* (Lindblom, 1959, 1979) or the *garbage can* model (van der Grinten, 1996:139). This bottom-up approach is inevitable in unstable, unpredictable situations with many actors, each with little power and little information—conditions found in a multicentric policy system. Not surprisingly, policy is not very important in this vision, as there is little scope for its design or implementation. Indeed, no formal policies may be stated (of course, these governments do have policies, but they are usually implicit[1]). Governments proceed by making small adjustments to past approaches, often in a piecemeal fashion. The minor adjustments reflect reality: there is rarely the opportunity to design a complex system from scratch, but it is often possible to make corrections to improve an existing system, e.g., by transferring a small amount of funding to exert a steering effect. And the little decisions can still be evidence based. But this policy model appears to be inefficient in that it can be extremely difficult to change direction or achieve goals. It has thus been seen as a highly conservative approach (Lindblom denies this), which tends to entrench the status quo. The United States and (lately) Canada exemplify this approach.

The characterization of the third, intermediate policy model is more variable, as is its fit with the pluricentric policy system. Dunn (1981: 230-1) refers to *bounded rationality* and to *constrained maximization,* which recognize that the capacity for rational decision making is limited. Other approaches focus on the complexity of the policy environment. Van der Grinten (1996:139) refers to a *mixed model,* which acknowledges that there are many rationalities that must be reconciled. The task of government is to organize communal decision making through extensive communication and negotiation, sometimes to the point of policy paralysis. Etzioni (1967) proposes *mixed scanning,* which uses both rational-comprehensive and incremental approaches, striving for the balance appropriate to each policy situation. Broad, strategic choices would alternate with incremental adjustments, based on detailed examination of narrower areas.

With some oversimplification, one might conclude that rational policy making is what ought to happen, incrementalism is what does happen,

[1]In response to a request for help in identifying Canadian health policy, the author was advised by a senior civil servant to undertake a content analysis of the health minister's speeches and press releases for the last 6 months, and draw his own conclusions.

and the variably named intermediate pattern might be something worth striving for. The complexity of the policymaking process should help the epidemiologist to understand why carefully formulated proposals are not automatically translated into policy: other factors are at work, as well as evidence. It is clear that policy is influenced by both evidence and politics, in varying proportions. Lindblom (1980:12) makes both sides of the argument: "[A]lthough the two main components of policymaking—analysis and politics—conflict with each other, they in some ways can complement each other." Richmond and Kotelchuck (1991) go further, suggesting that successful introduction of policy depends upon (1) an adequate knowledge base, (2) political will, and (3) a social strategy (e.g., the Healthy People initiative in the U.S.). This book aims to show the epidemiologist how to contribute to the evidence and understand a little of the politics.

1.4 The Policy Cycle

Policymaking is a continuing and iterative process, suggesting a cyclical structure. This facilitates organized thinking about policy, even if the actual process is often less orderly. Several cyclical models with varying numbers of steps are presented here, to illustrate the diversity in approaches and provide a range of ideas.

Walt (1994:45) presents four stages for the policy process:

1. Problem identification and issue recognition
2. Policy formulation
3. Policy implementation
4. Policy evaluation.

Dutch health policy also follows a four-step cycle, but starts with evaluation, recognizing that there is almost always relevant existing policy (Ruwaard et al., 1994:22):

1. Policy evaluation
2. Policy preparation
3. Policy development
4. Policy implementation.

Policy evaluation compares developments in health status with the government's current health objectives. *Policy preparation* concerns the overall thrust of future policy and formulation of alternative proposals, and is to occur every 3–4 years. *Policy development* elaborates selected proposals, considering issues like funding, and is to occur every year, in some cases every 3–4 years. *Policy implementation* includes legislation and regulations along with direct programming. Epidemiology contributes mainly to steps 1 and 2 of the cycle, in the form of a *Public Health Status and Forecasts* report, issued once per cycle and an outstanding example of the applica-

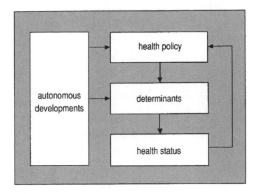

Figure 1-1. Conceptual model for health policy making. [From Ruwaard et al., 1994:29, with permission.]

tion of epidemiology to health policy. The underlying conceptual model is shown in Figure 1-1.

Dunn (1981:48) presents an integrated framework (shown in Fig. 1-2), showing both the steps in the cycle and the contributions of various policy analytic techniques (discussed below). He acknowledges that in practice the components are not always linked in exactly this way.

In contrast, Barker's (1996:28) policy process has seven elements (Fig. 1-3). Although goals (see Section 7.1) may sometimes be defined at this

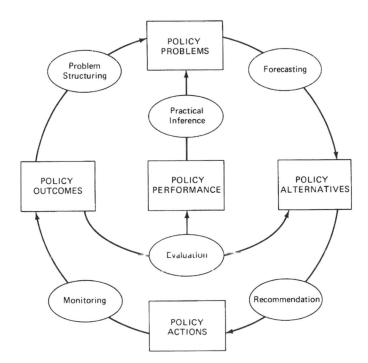

Figure 1-2. The process of policy analysis. [From Dunn, 1981:48, with permission.]

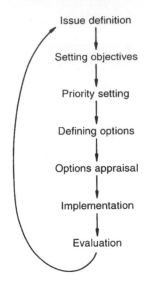

Figure 1-3. Stages in the policymaking process. [Reprinted by permission of Sage Publications Ltd. from Barker C., The Health Policy Process, Copyright (Carol Barker 1996).]

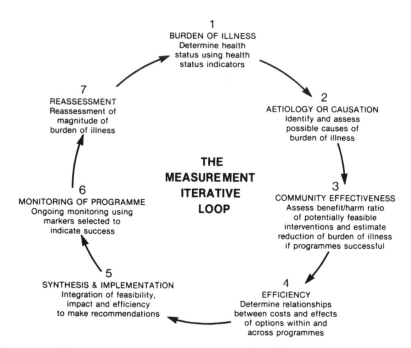

Figure 1-4. The measurement iterative loop. [Reprinted from Journal of Chronic Diseases, 38, Tugwell P, Bennett KJ, Sackett DL, Haynes RB, The Measurement Iterative Loop: a framework for the critical appraisal of need, benefits and costs of health interventions, pp. 339–51, Copyright (1985), with permission from Elsevier Science.]

early stage, it is hard to see how objectives, which should be attainable and must be measurable, can be formulated until after consideration of the available interventions. Options appraisal often includes scenario development.

The *measurement iterative loop* was developed by Tugwell et al. (1985: 339) as "a framework for assembling the specific subset of health information that is most likely to tell us how to reduce the burden of both morbidity and mortality." This process, summarized in Figure 1-4, is intended to guide approaches to a specific health problem. As discussed in Section 5.3, the very useful concept of community effectiveness is defined as the product of efficacy, diagnostic accuracy, provider compliance, patient compliance, and coverage.

Finally, Mayer and Greenwood (1980:8–12) present the nine-stage process shown in Figure 1-5, noting that the first three steps might occur in

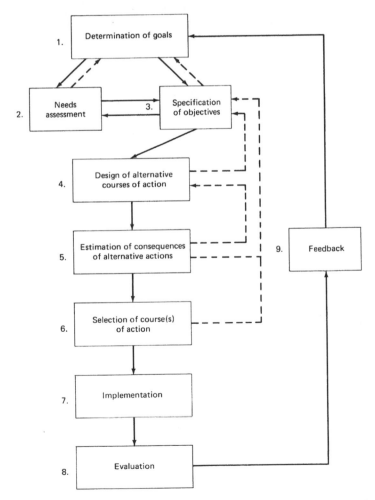

Figure 1-5. Flow of stages in the policymaking process. [From Mayer and Greenwood, 1980:9, with permission.]

various sequences. The internal feedback loops further recognize that policymaking is not always a linear process.

The Policy Cycle Used Here

The cycle shown in Figure 1-6 will serve as the organizing framework for Part II of this book. The cycle has been restricted to a fairly small number of steps. Some policy cycles include an agenda-setting step, which considers how issues come to be considered as possible topics for policy development. This step is replaced here by identification of health problems and needs, since of the many routes by which topics get on the policy agenda, these are the ones to which epidemiology can contribute. Designing alternative courses of action, estimating their consequences, and selecting one or more courses for implementation have been combined into the single step of making policy choices. Specification of goals has been seen as primarily the policymaker's prerogative, while specification of objectives has been seen from the epidemiologists' perspective as a tool for implementation and evaluation. The cycle is admittedly idealized, in that some steps may sometimes be undertaken in different sequence or even omitted. For example, it is widely acknowledged that implementation influences policymaking, so the relation between the two is reciprocal (Lindblom, 1980:65; Walt, 1994:156). It will become apparent that epidemiology can make significant contributions to every step of the cycle.

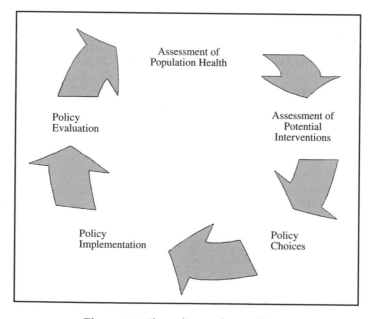

Figure 1-6. The policy cycle used here.

Policy and Programs

Policies define goals and the broad approaches that will be used to achieve them. But they need to be turned into actions if they are to have any effect. The actual policy instruments for implementing policy are listed by Pal (1992:143) as follows:

- *Nodality*: the quality of being in the center of information networks, e.g., through responding to queries or disseminating information, or through exhortation and consultation, to which might be added such tactics as delay and changing priorities and decisions regarding how rigorously to enforce legislation and regulations)
- *Treasure*: spending power, as exerted through grants, subsidies, insurance and tax incentives, and purchasing practices
- *Authority*: control measures including legislation, public regulation, self-regulation, and sanctions
- *Organization*: government operations through direct provision of services, public corporations, or partnerships.

Any of these instruments might be called a *health program*, although that term is often used to refer specifically to direct provision of services. Even this narrower usage can refer either to a program concept, e.g., home care, or to a specific implementation of the concept, e.g., the home care program in a specific city. Whatever the usage, programs exist within the framework of policy, and are influenced and constrained by it. There is a rather similar program cycle that operates within the policy implementation step of the policy cycle, but this book does not directly address program planning and evaluation. In fact, the distinction between policies and programs is not always perfectly clear (see next section); much of the material in this book applies to both.

1.5 Policy Studies

A number of intellectual activities are more or less closely related to health policy, several of them being relatively new and most of them (given the complexity of the policy environment) multidisciplinary.

Policy analysis has become an important multidisciplinary field, comprising the research and development arm of policy. Its boundaries are not very clearly defined. According to Dunn (1981:35), "policy analysis is an applied social science discipline which uses multiple methods of inquiry and argument to produce and transform policy-relevant information that may be utilized in political settings to resolve policy problems." Pal (1992:16) offers a broader but briefer definition: "the disciplined application of intellect to public problems." Since it focuses on broad questions and on the future, policy analysis is subject to considerable uncertainty. Policy analysis usually draws on existing research, expert judgment, and deductive modeling, but does not include the conduct of empirical research (Shortell and Solomon, 1982). By any of these definitions, this text concerns the contribution of epidemiology to policy analysis. Dunn (1981:38–41) identifies three broad approaches and six specific analytical procedures used in policy analysis; these are summarized in Table 1-1. The *empirical* approach is concerned with facts and includes both monitoring the past effects of policies (description) and forecasting their future effects (prediction). The *evaluative* approach is concerned with values, as the word suggests; the corresponding procedure can apply to both past and (through modeling) future policies. The *normative* approach comprises recommendations for future actions (prescription). Two more general procedures apply to all approaches and times: *problem structuring* or asking the right question, which is central to the whole process, and *practical inference* or drawing conclusions from social values and norms as well as empirical results. In principle, the procedures lead to a *policy argument* (Dunn, 1981:40–3), which should include policy-relevant background, a policy claim or recommendation, justification for the claim, and necessary qualifiers.

Health policy research is complementary to policy analysis, comprising original investigations of narrower questions, thus focusing mostly on the past. *Health services research* examines operational details of more interest to managers and practitioners, but often provides important support for health policy analysis.

Health technology assessment initially referred to clinical and economic evaluation of technological innovations in medicine, especially very expensive ones. But the field has expanded to encompass comprehensive studies of both new and old, and both large and small, technologies, which even include the physical examination. Medical technology includes "the drugs, devices, and medical and surgical procedures used in medical care, and the organization and supportive systems within which such care is provided. . . . Technology assessment [is] a comprehensive form of policy research that examines the technical, economic, and social consequences of technological applications. It is especially concerned with unintended, indirect, or delayed social impacts. In health policy, the

Table 1-1. Analytical Procedures in Policy Analysis

Time	Approach (Concern)		
	Empirical (Facts)	**Evaluative (Values)**	**Normative (Actions)**
Before action	Prediction	Evaluation (modeling)	Prescription
After action	Description	Evaluation	—

Source: Table adapted from Dunn (1981:37,39), with permission

term has also come to mean any form of policy analysis concerned with medical technology, especially the evaluation of efficacy and safety" (U.S. Congress, 1982:200–2). For many practitioners, health technology assessment is therefore almost synonymous with health care policy analysis (Goodman, 1992).

Health planning (health program planning, health services planning) is closely related to policy, and some people make little distinction between them. For example, Mayer and Greenwood (1980:6) use the terms interchangeably, although they sometimes distinguish between policy planning and program planning. Indeed, the two activities share many information needs. But other authorities see planning as a lower-level activity, conducted within the framework of policy: "planning follows policy: planners help to put policies into practice, although the planning process itself may help to develop and refine health policies" (Walt, 1994: 7).

The term *public health* appears to have at least two distinct uses (Ruwaard et al., 1994:28). The *Dictionary of Epidemiology* (Last, 1995:134) defines it as "the combination of science, skills, and beliefs that is directed to the maintenance and improvement of the health of all the people through collective or social actions." Similarly, the Acheson report in the United Kingdom (Commission of Inquiry, 1988) saw public health as "the science and art of preventing disease, prolonging life and promoting health through organized efforts of society." This conforms to common usage of the term in North America and Britain for the package of direct services normally provided by government agencies; but does it also include health services planning or state health insurance? The content of major textbooks on public health (Detels et al., 1997; Last and Wallace, 1992) and of the *Journal of Public Health Policy* suggests that these activities are included under the rubric public health, although they are usually conducted quite separately from public health practice. Thus, public health and health policy are much intertwined. In continental Europe, public health often appears to refer to the health of the public, e.g., "the extent and spread of diseases, disability and mortality in the population" (van der Maas et al., 1989, as translated in Ruwaard et al., 1994:28). Perhaps slightly preciously, this concept is sometimes referred to as "the public's health" or even "*the* public health." For our purposes, the *Dictionary* definition cited above will be used here.

Population health is a newer term (it does not appear in the third edition of the *Dictionary of Epidemiology*), which sometimes appears to have roughly the same two meanings as public health, but with special emphasis placed on the social and economic determinants of health (Evans et al., 1994). Hayes and Dunn (1998) distinguish among population health as a perspective, an area of research, a conceptual framework, and an approach to health policy, the first approach subsuming the other three. All of these approaches emphasize the health of the entire population of a country or region, not just the users of health services, or other subgroups.

1.6 Epidemiology and Health Policy

Policymakers need information on what is currently happening, what is likely to happen in the future in the absence of interventions, and what is likely to happen in the presence of interventions. This includes information on determinants and trends in health, and the implications of changes in health. Generation of this information requires contributions from several social sciences, e.g., demography, geography, and economics, as well as the biological and medical sciences, especially epidemiology.

Contribution of Epidemiology to Health Policy

This book attempts to show how epidemiology can contribute to the policy process and thus to "evidence-based policymaking" (Muir Gray, 1997). Many factors influence policy, and it can be hard to find examples where policy has been influenced by research results. Sometimes the problem is looking for very direct links; more often, science exerts its influence through a broader process of "enlightenment" of policymakers (Walt, 1994:181). Holland and Wainwright (1979) provide numerous examples of cases in which the results of epidemiology have influenced health policy, but they concede that there is often a long time lag before this occurs, and that a further 5–10 years may pass before such policy decisions can be evaluated. Epidemiologists should thus recognize the policy system and model that are in place, and adapt their work to that model; there is no use making grand plans if the system will not accommodate them, and no use communicating with the wrong people. What is the nature of contributions from epidemiology? Four main headings spring to mind: a population focus, health and prevention, health services, and health information.

Population focus.

Public policy concerns actions that affect populations. As "the study of the distribution and determinants of health-related states or events in specified populations, and the application of this study to control of health problems" (Last, 1995:55), epidemiology is well positioned to maintain a population perspective, balancing the clinician's emphasis on individuals. Policy epidemiology is always projected on to a real-world population. Indeed, for policy purposes, the size and characteristics of a population are as important as the rates at which health events and states occur within it. Thus, a health problem may be frequent because its sector-specific incidence rate is high or because the segment of the population that it affects is large. This interrelation of numerator and denominator factors pervades all of policy epidemiology and makes demography an essential sister discipline. The emphasis on projecting the findings on to the population makes the external validity of research findings as important as their internal validity, and the distribution of exposures and interventions as important as their effects. The contribution of epidemiology is complementary to that of other population-oriented disciplines, such as economics (especially analysis of health-care costs, and value for money spent), social psychology (determinants of health behavior), and ethics (public values).

Health and prevention.

The contribution of epidemiology goes well beyond the findings of etiological research. Epidemiology can help to maintain the centrality of health outcomes in the policy process, as distinct from health services utilization or financial outcomes (Ibrahim, 1985:5–6). Similarly, Terris (1980) suggests that a health policy based on epidemiology would have as its major goal the development of programs to prevent the major causes of death. Kuller (1988) divides diseases into seven categories on the basis of how much is known about their cause and treatment, and defines the contribution of epidemiology to each group, ranging from descriptive and etiologic studies of those about which least is known, to program surveillance and public health education for those whose care is well defined. But he also identifies an advocacy role: "The critical challenge to public health policy is to narrow the socioeconomic gradient in morbidity and mortality and to encourage more positive health behaviors in the total population" (Kuller, 1988:14).

Health services.

Epidemiology has a major role in monitoring the quality and quantity of health care, especially in measuring health outcomes and conducting evaluations. Noting that quality of health care is usually measured as structure, process, or outcome, and that quantity is related to utilization and costs, Kuller (1988:2) argues that "the further introduction of epidemiologic methods into health policy analysis will reduce costs and improve the quality of health care." He goes on to acknowledge the differing perspectives of politicians, professionals, public health advocates, and consumers, and suggests (rather ambitiously) that "one goal of the epidemiologist in health planning is to try to synthesize these varied health policy views." (Kuller, 1988:6)

Health information.

Policymakers deal continually with uncertainty, and epidemiology can help to reduce that uncertainty and define its boundaries. Epidemiology can contribute both kinds of health information needed for health policy making: (1) descriptive information on the health of the population and the utilization of health services, and (2) analytical information on the causes of health problems and the effectiveness of health services. Clinical epidemiologists have developed systematic approaches to assessing and synthesizing such evidence and resolving the frequent conflicts that it contains. Shapiro (1991) addresses both categories of evidence by suggesting that the contribution of epidemiology is twofold: to identify determinants of health and to conduct systematic monitoring. He argues that the most important direct impact of epidemiology has been the information it has produced on the magnitude of health problems and risk factors and on prevention and control of health conditions, but that we need still better information and in particular, need to integrate data from routine information systems with data from research projects. He cites the Healthy People initiative (Department of Health and Human Services, 1991) and the Guide to Clinical Preventive Services (U.S. Preventive Services Task Force, 1996) as examples of the constructive application of epidemiology to health policy.

How do these general contributions relate to the stages in the policy cycle? It is worth going through them systematically.

Epidemiology and the policy cycle

1. Assessment of population health (Chap. 4). Epidemiologists can contribute to the conceptualization and measurement of health, using their expertise in population health data. More particularly, they can assess health needs and risks, determine the impact of health problems on society, and examine inequalities in health. Most epidemiologic research is devoted to determining the causes of health and health problems; study of population-level determinants is especially relevant to policy.

2. Assessment of potential interventions (Chap. 5). Epidemiologists can evaluate and synthesize the evidence regarding the efficacy of potential interventions and can assess their likely effectiveness.

3. Policy choices (Chap. 6). Epidemiologists can advise on the potential for preventing diseases, model the impact of various interventions on the overall health of the population, and provide an objective basis to help select priorities from among the options.

4. Policy implementation (Chap. 7). Epidemiologists can contribute to the setting of meaningful goals and objectives, provide a rational basis for resource allocation, and advise on the data that will be needed to support policy evaluation.

5. Policy evaluation (Chap. 8). Epidemiologists can assist in developing a rigorous evaluation design, and can conduct surveillance of health problems and health services, detecting unusual occurrences and evaluating small area variations in health care.

Which Epidemiologic Methods?

Epidemiology has absorbed methods from a wide range of disciplines, including demography, geography, and the social sciences, and has developed its own methods for studying the health of populations. Mainstream epidemiology, especially in North America, focuses on etiological research, and thus emphasizes analytical epidemiology. As summarized in Table 1-2, the contributions of epidemiology to health policy often

Table 1-2. Types of Epidemiology

Dimension	Etiologic Epidemiology	Policy Epidemiology
Approach	Analytical	Usually descriptive; modeling
Purpose	Find causes	Guide policy
Activities	Research projects	Research synthesis and application
Data	New (specially collected)	Existing (often administrative)
Substrate	Samples	Whole populations
Time reference	Past	Future
Validity emphasis	Internal	Internal and external
Clients	Scientists, practitioners	Governments, decision makers

come from descriptive epidemiology, which appears to occupy a rather low status in the discipline. Estève et al. (1994) provide a long-overdue treatment of descriptive epidemiology, providing it with a firm methodologic foundation. The results of analytical epidemiologic research are equally relevant to policy, but require some adaptation for that purpose. Analytical epidemiology is conducted in carefully selected samples, with a view to determining the effect of an exposure, whereas policy epidemiology is more concerned with the impact of the exposure on the general population and more often with the prediction than the explanation of health phenomena. Relevant methods appear in Chapter 2. Policy is often based on aggregated data, either because this is preferable (where variables act at the population level) or because no information on individuals is available, whereas etiologic researchers usually and clinicians always prefer individual data. The different data call for quite different methods, which are discussed in Chapters 3 and 4. Two other differences do not require special methods, but they do imply a different emphasis from mainstream epidemiology.

The first is the importance of raw numbers. A basic principle of mainstream epidemiology, with its emphasis on etiological research, is that numbers of events are rarely interpretable until converted to rates. But this principle does not necessarily apply to policy studies. When the burden of ill health or the needs for health care of a population are being assessed, the absolute number of cases of or deaths from a condition is more relevant than the rate (epidemiology's devotion to denominators need not suffer, since it is crucial that the population from which the cases arose be defined).

The other emphasis in policy-oriented epidemiologic analysis is the importance of crude rates. Crude (unstandardized) rates have great utility for health policy, and for similar reasons. If a population is relatively old and has the high prevalence of chronic disease or disability associated with advanced age, then that high prevalence is relevant for estimating the burden of ill health that the population suffers, determining needs, and planning services. Age standardization would remove the effect of age and thereby conceal the magnitude of the population's problems and needs; crude rates will be more valuable. Of course, if the objective is to explain the high prevalence of health problems or to assess the healthfulness of living conditions in various areas, then standardized rates are essential.

Most textbooks and journals of epidemiology focus on epidemiologic research, but two recent textbooks address topics more relevant to health policy. The text edited by Armenian and Shapiro (1998) introduces epidemiology to health services managers, while that edited by Brownson and Petitti (1998) prepares epidemiologists to work in the public health sector. Relevant articles are more often found in journals of public health, including the *Journal of Epidemiology and Community Health*, the *Journal of Public Health Policy*, and especially *Annual Review of Public Health*, and journals on health care, such as *Medical Care*, *Health Services Research*, and the *Journal of Health Politics, Policy and Law* than in mainstream epidemiology journals.

Limitations of Epidemiology

Many authors have deplored the fact that epidemiology is not well used in decision making, despite its potential. The reasons relate to both epidemiologists and policymakers.

For their part, epidemiologic researchers do not address the questions for which policymakers need answers, take too long to do their work, and do not promulgate their results in venues that policymakers will see or in forms that policymakers can understand. Many observers (e.g., Brownson, 1998) have noted the increasing isolation of academic epidemiology far from public health and policy operations and thus from real problems. Others have criticized the discipline's whole paradigm. Levine and Lilienfeld (1987:3) note that "epidemiologists are still struggling to free themselves of the older model of a single etiological agent producing a specific disease," and Stallones (1980:75) claims that "the most complicated [mathematical] models are simplistic by comparison with the social and biological realities, and the judgments required are too subtle to be reduced to a set of rules or a mathematical expression" (perhaps this is an argument for wider use of qualitative methods). Similarly, social scientists have argued that public health, traditional epidemiology and other health services researchers address these issues inadequately because they adhere to the biomedical model of health. Omenn (1993) addresses the limitations of epidemiologic research on environmental hazards, particularly the fact that results are seldom definitive, and the difficulty of proving a negative result. He calls for closer interaction with toxicology and improved risk communication skills.

On the other hand, policymakers may not understand research, often demand immediate results, and cannot tolerate uncertainty. Health professionals and society have failed to understand the primacy of prevention, being unwilling to accept the validity of epidemiologic discoveries and too subject to the power of private interests (Terris, 1980).

More fundamental than the deficiencies of either party is simply the imperfect fit between the two. Health-policy makers need clear advice based on available data, whereas epidemiologists prefer interval estimates (rather than simple answers or yes–no decisions) and multiple empirical studies (instead of a single quick-and-dirty study). Syme and Guralik (1987) ascribe the complicated path from epidemiology to public policy to (1) differences in the interpretation of evidence; (2) differences in the priority given to various specific interventions; and (3) differences regarding whether interventions should be at the individual or community level. They refer to the work of Winkelstein and Marmot (1981) regarding whether prevention should follow a medical model (preventive interventions by doctors and other health professionals), a public health model (health education and community organization directed at entire communities), or an ecological model (structural changes in the community). They also note (pp. 111–2) the differing priorities of the two fields: "While it would be of value to continue the search for new risk factors, it is perhaps even more important at this time to use epidemiologic tools to determine optimal ways of reducing known risk factors."

Is Policy Epidemiology Research?

Policy epidemiology is indeed research, in that it is "a systematic process for generating new knowledge" (Walt 1994:178). The topics are more immediately relevant to society than those of most etiologic research, and the linkage to decision makers is much more direct. Indeed, the topics will often be supplied by the decision maker. The demands that this research makes for methodologic expertise are as great as those of etiologic research, although different and broader, drawing from many other disciplines. The demands for creativity are also great, although less for hypothesis formulation than for creative resolutions to problems, finding compromises, and determining what sorts of evidence presented in what ways are most likely to lead to beneficial policies.

1.7 Ethics and Advocacy

A recent volume edited by Coughlin and Beauchamp (1996) comprehensively reviews ethical issues in epidemiology, with emphasis on etiological research. Although policy epidemiology rarely involves even making observations on individuals (much less manipulating them), the activities of epidemiologists working on health policy may have greater ethical implications than etiological research. Epidemiologists' values can influence their approach to health problems, e.g., whether to focus on diseases or on population groups, or to address physiological, behavioral, or environmental risk factors. The indicators that epidemiologists use to measure some construct will reflect their particular view of the world, just as the values (utilities) placed on various health states when calculating quality-adjusted life years (QALYs) will ultimately place a greater or lesser value on various groups in society. There is no way that these influences can be eliminated; this work is not value-free.

Generic ethical principles (Last, 1994) apply to policy epidemiology. *Autonomy* includes respect for privacy, which is often the biggest issue for epidemiologists, but is perhaps less critical for those working in policy than for those doing etiologic research, who must frequently review the records of individuals. *Beneficence* requires that actions be expected to benefit the participants and requires careful attention to evidence of effectiveness and optimal use of resources. The principle of *non-maleficence*, that actions should not harm the participants, may be less frequently relevant to epidemiology than to clinical practice, but some programs, e.g., screening programs, have definite potential to do harm. *Justice* refers to a fair distribution of risks and benefits, and epidemiology can influence this through its participation in setting goals and priorities and in allocating resources; e.g., should the emphasis be on equity or efficiency?.

Epidemiologists and users of their results should be aware of these issues and should expose their values and assumptions. Important research decisions should be taken by broadly representative groups, generally including consumers, rather than by the epidemiologist alone. Sensitivity analyses should be conducted, addressing questions like, "Suppose that we had valued a particular health state 30% higher; then what would have emerged as a priority?."

Codes of ethics promulgated by general research agencies may fail to recognize the peculiarities of epidemiologic research, especially the distinction between physically invasive techniques and interviewing, and the epidemiologist's need to use data collected for another purpose (without having any interest in the identity of the individuals). Specialized codes of ethics have been developed for epidemiologic research (Council for International Organizations of Medical Sciences, 1991).

The Epidemiologist as Policy Advocate

When epidemiologists do policy-relevant work, they can hope to see their results reflected in policy. It is their ethical responsibility to communicate their results effectively to policymakers and perhaps to the general public. But effective communication may shade into political advocacy, and this may lead to trouble, or at least controversy. For instance, during the planning for the First Canadian Epidemiology and Biostatistics Conference some years ago, there was a sharp polarization between those members of the planning committee who argued that a session on epidemiology and health policy was essential (all of whom happened to be health-professional epidemiologists) and those who argued that epidemiologists should stick to pure science (none of whom happened to be health-professional epidemiologists). Rothman and Poole (1985:341) argue that "the conduct of science should be guided by the pursuit of explanations for natural phenomena, not the attainment of political or social objectives." On the other hand, Weed (1994) concludes that advocacy is justified by existing ethical codes, and even becomes a necessity when dealing with prevention. The journal *Epidemiology* prohibits epidemiologists from making policy recommendations in scientific articles, requiring that these be presented in editorials, letters, and commentaries (Rothman, 1993). Its reasons are that policy is too difficult to be tossed out lightly in the form of recommendations at the end of a paper, and that authors may be overly influenced by their own research findings. Not surprisingly, the policy provoked a vigorous debate (Teret, 1993; Coughlin, 1994; Dietz-Rioux et al., 1994). In contrast, this book is for epidemiologists working in or with the policy sector, whose job it is to make policy recommendations.

The Epidemiologist in Government

The epidemiologist in government is in a particularly sensitive position. The employer's permission may be needed before publishing a scientific paper. This can be highly problematic when the epidemiologist discovers specific health problems that the government may wish to suppress, or holds views inconsistent with government policy (e.g., regarding tobacco policy). Some government epidemiologists have found it useful to develop a continuing collaboration with colleagues from outside government, allowing the outsider to take the lead on delicate issues. In a few cases the epidemiologist may have to decide whether to become a whistle-blower or leaker of privileged information in plain brown envelopes, or to seek other employment. But the excellent work done in many countries by government-employed epidemiologists suggests that such drastic measures are rarely needed. Much of this work is cited throughout this book.

1.8 Legal Issues: Access to Data and Protection of Privacy

Policy-relevant epidemiology often requires access to sensitive data files, e.g., for conduct of computerized record linkage. The agencies that hold data relevant to public health workers have a legal responsibility to protect the privacy of the persons to whom the data relate. They therefore establish rules regarding when data will be released and which specific figures will be suppressed, to ensure that individuals cannot be identified. Although public health workers are not interested in data on individuals, they are frequently very interested in small areas, and the rules can limit their ability to produce the detailed pictures that they desire (and that policymakers need). Although this situation can be frustrating, small sample sizes can make the data for these small areas unreliable, so the privacy provisions actually protect the epidemiologist from drawing unsupportable conclusions. Agencies concerned with protection of privacy have been highly critical of the use of health records for purposes other than those for which they were originally collected, especially in computerized record linkage studies (see Chap. 3), and it has been difficult to persuade such agencies that the benefits often outweigh the costs. The European Community at one point proposed regulations that would virtually stop epidemiologic research, although its revised proposals are less extreme (Olsen, 1995; Lynge, 1995).

1.9 Communication Skills

The epidemiologist's work cannot influence policy unless it is adequately communicated. Although not generally taught in epidemiology graduate programs, communication skills are often as important as technical research skills. This applies not only to the epidemiologist working in government but also to other epidemiologists who wish their work to influence policy. While much policy epidemiology work is done in response to a request (e.g., instructions from an employer, a contract with government), nongovernmental epidemiologists must practice "proactive" communication with policymakers and media. A particularly thorny problem is dealing with conflicting evidence, often arising from relatively small studies of weak associations—associations that have much policy relevance but results that offer no clear guidance. Thorough treatment of this issue is provided by Dan (1996) and Remington (1998).

Communicating with Policymakers

As noted above, senior health-policymakers often have little understanding of health issues and know even less about epidemiology. In order to influence policy, the epidemiologist must understand how the policy process works; who the policymakers are; what information they need, and when; what other input the policymakers will receive; and how best to communicate with them.

Articles in professional journals are certainly not the best way to communicate with policy-makers, but policy papers, briefs, and briefings may be. Some points to consider are the following:

- *Language* used should avoid epidemiologic or medical jargon and especially mathematics, and explain concepts in plain English.
- *Graphics* aid communication; maps are especially effective. Detailed data can go into an appendix.
- *Examples* are easier to understand than expository text or formulas, especially examples relevant to the policymaker's own experience.
- *Relevance* is crucial. Relate the material to the population for which the policymaker is responsible, e.g., "We estimate that the policy could prevent 800 deaths in your area every year."

- *Brevity* increases the probability of the report being read. Summaries of 1–2 pages are essential.

An epidemiologist working on health policy will frequently have to produce *policy issue papers* to structure policy problems for policymakers. Dunn (1981:363) provides an outline for such a paper that recapitulates the policy cycle and is based on the analytic procedures he identifies. Such a paper should begin with a letter of transmittal and an executive summary, and the body of the paper should contain the following elements:

1. The source and background of the *problematic situation* including its description, outcomes of prior efforts, an assessment of past policy performance, and the significance of the situation.
2. The *policy problem*, which includes statement of the problem, the approach to analysis, identification of major stakeholders and of goals and objectives, measures of effectiveness, and potential solutions.
3. Policy *alternatives*. These are presented through description and comparison, and address spillovers and externalities, constraints, and political feasibility.
4. Policy *recommendations* include criteria for recommending alternatives, a description of preferred alternative(s), an outline of implementation strategy, provisions for monitoring and evaluation, limitations and unanticipated consequences.

Finally, the policy issue paper should conclude with references and appendices. Dunn also provides a checklist of 30 questions for use in preparing such papers (Dunn, 1981:364).

In most policy systems, the range of policymakers is very wide. As in addressing the media (discussed below), a continuing communications strategy allows the epidemiologist to learn how policymakers think and what they want; this strategy is likely to be more successful than sporadic efforts.

Communicating with the Media

Health policy is of great interest to the media because health is a politically and emotionally hot topic. This interest extends to the work of epidemiologists, especially with regard to environmental factors in disease causation. There is a certain amount of built-in tension between epidemiologists and the media, much of it resulting from difficulties in the reporting and interpretation of weak associations in causal research. From the standpoint of the epidemiologist, it may appear as though the media

- are interested only in spectacular new "cures" and "breakthroughs" in biomedical science, not in causes or prevention;

- do not understand that research results are subject to error;
- expect results immediately, without recognition of the time that research takes;
- want only an 8-second clip for the evening television news, and are not interested in understanding complicated issues.

From the standpoint of the media, epidemiologists

- have no sense of time;
- are more interested in the ways that evidence might be wrong than in the evidence itself;
- cannot speak intelligible English;
- may be primarily interested in furthering their own academic careers.

The issues have been well played out in a famous article by Taubes (1995) in *Science* and in the ensuing debates in several journals (e.g., Wynder, 1996). Attitudes are important; the epidemiologist should remember that journalist' are simply doing their job and that they have an important role to play in a democratic society.

All of the communications skills mentioned earlier will have a place in media relations. Some additional guidelines for communication with the media are provided by Altman et al. (1994:105–15):

1. Practice *Targeting:* find the right persons to talk to (usually the science or medical writers) and develop a lasting professional relationship with those persons to develop their expertise and to build up an atmosphere of trust.
2. Use *press conferences* (but not often enough to bore the media), prepare well, and make only a few key points.
3. Use *press releases*, providing a summary of the important issues and showing why they are important.

Summary

Policy is a set of standing principles used to guide decisions. It provides guideposts against which to test proposals and ideas, and a framework within which program planning and evaluation can occur. Any set of consistent decisions is based on policy, even if that policy is not explicit. Public policy is the policies of governments. Governments exhibit several different approaches to policy, ranging from the rational-deductive approach of planned economies to the incrementalism of some western nations, with mixed scanning being an alternative approach that tries to combine the best qualities of both. Health policy refers to all policy intended to influence health; it may address health determinants, public health, or personal health care. This book is concerned mainly with public health policy, which is public policy concerning health. Ideally, the policy process forms a cycle, beginning with assessment of health problems and of potential interventions and proceeding to policy choices, followed by implementation and evaluation. But reality is rarely this tidy. Epidemiology can be used to provide a population focus for policy analysis, contribute expert knowledge of prevention, contribute to the study of health services, and provide and interpret health information. The most relevant epidemiologic methods are often drawn from descriptive epidemiology, which is relatively neglected in most textbooks. Policy epidemiology can be intellectually stimulating and rigorous, although the research topics are provided externally, along with challenging deadlines. Health policies are developed and implemented in an environment of conflicting pressures. The values of the epidemiologist can influence the work, e.g., in terms of selection of variables and concepts. Ways must be found to acknowledge and compensate for this influence, e.g., through obtaining broad input (especially from the public) and conducting sensitivity analyses. The work will frequently involve use and linkage of sensitive data files, necessitating protection of privacy. The epidemiologist in government is in a particularly sensitive position, and may encounter conflicts between personal values and those of the employer. In addition to appropriate methodologic expertise, the epidemiologist working in policy must possess skills in communication and must understand enough of related disciplines to work effectively with them. Relationships with the media can be as delicate as those with the policymakers.

Key References

Dunn WN. *Public Policy. An Introduction.* Englewood Cliffs, NJ: Prentice-Hall, 1981.

Ibrahim M. *Epidemiology and Health Policy.* Rockville, MD: Aspen Systems Corporation, 1985.

Levine S, Lilienfeld A (eds). *Epidemiology and Health Policy.* New York and London: Tavistock Publications, 1987.

Walt G. *Health Policy. An Introduction to Process and Power.* London: Zed Books, 1994.

2

Some Tools of the Trade

Most textbooks of epidemiologic methods focus on etiological research and thus on analytical designs. This chapter addresses three areas, drawn from demography, clinical epidemiology and health economics, and population epidemiology, that are highly relevant to policy but are relatively neglected in standard textbooks. Material that is well covered in conventional textbooks is for the most part not duplicated here.

2.1 Demography and Vital Statistics

Analytical epidemiology deals with associations between exposures and outcomes, and usually has little concern for the populations in which these epidemiologic phenomena occur. But policy occurs in society, making population directly relevant, so demography and vital statistics are important topics for health policy.

Natality

The most common statistic for natality is the (crude) *live birth rate,* but this statistic suffers from the same problems as those of the crude death rate in that both are strongly affected by the age and sex composition of the population. A high or low rate may simply reflect the presence of many or few women of reproductive age, and have nothing to do with reproductive behavior or performance. Age-standardized birth rates are rarely calculated, but age- and sex-specific rates are commonly used, in the form of measures of fertility.

Fertility

Fertility is important for health policy because it is the main determinant of the population's age composition and because it tends to change quickly and unpredictably. Measures of fertility relate the number of births to the female population of reproductive age, thus providing the most useful measure of reproductive performance. Several variants exist, including

$$\text{(General) Fertility Rate} = \frac{\text{Number of Live Births during a Year}}{\text{Mid-year Population of Women aged 15--44 Years}} \times 1000$$

The fertility rate can also be calculated on an age-specific basis, normally for 5-year age-groups:

$$\text{Age-specific Fertility Rate (aged } x) = \frac{\text{Live Births to Women Aged } x}{\text{Mid-year Population of Women Aged } x} \times 1000$$

The sum of the age-specific fertility rates over the entire reproductive span is the *total fertility rate* (Peron and Strohmenger, 1985: 72–5), which is the number of live births that a cohort of women would have during their entire reproductive span if current age-specific fertility rates were to continue (the same assumption as made in a period life table). In the steady state, i.e., no changes in age-specific fertility over time, this equals the *completed fertility rate*, which is the total number of live births per female (Peron and Strohmenger, 1985: 41–5). The rate is currently around 1.7 in North America, well below the replacement level of 2.1, but the rate of natural increase remains positive because there are still so many young women in the population—an illustration of the importance of demographic structure in determining the frequency of events.

Mortality

Mortality is most often expressed by the death rate, which may be crude or standardized (adjusted), and general (all causes) or cause-specific. The *absolute number of deaths* and the *crude death rate* are often most useful for policy purposes, as direct measures of one type of event with which the health care system must deal. Three other concepts require more discussion: potential years of life lost, life tables, and fatality.

Potential years of life lost

Numbers and rates of deaths are useful information, but a better measure of the impact of a disease on the population is the *potential years of life lost* (PYLL), in which the age of each decedent from the disease is subtracted from some "normal" age of death, and the total accumulated:

$$\text{PYLL} = \Sigma \text{ ("Normal" Age for Death – Actual Age at Death)}$$

In the past, deaths in the first year of life were often omitted, on the grounds that they have quite different causes and require different preventive interventions from those occurring after infancy. The usual practice at present is to include infant deaths in the calculation. Like numbers of deaths, PYLL can be expressed as rates (crude or specific) and can be age standardized; this is important, for the overall PYLL is as affected by the age composition of the population as the crude death rate is. The PYLL may be calculated for all causes of death or for specific causes. The calculations usually ignore competing risks (see below): one does not actually know how long a person would have lived if she or he had not died from a specific cause.

Any such calculation gives less weight to diseases occurring later in life (e.g., stroke) than to those occurring in childhood, but the specific results depend upon the age defined as "normal" for death. The standard retirement age of 65 has been most used, but with the graying of the population the cutoff has been edging up to as high as 85. The life expectancy at the age of death can be used to estimate *expected years of life lost* (EYLL), although this complicates comparisons among different jurisdictions or times, as life expectancies vary. Murray (1994) reviews the calculation of PYLL (based on a fixed limit), *period EYLL* (from a period life table), *cohort EYLL* (from a cohort life table), and *standard EYLL* (from an "ideal" life table, e.g., the best national experience, currently that of Japan). All of these measures are gradually being replaced by disability-adjusted life years (DALYs) or other methods incorporating some measure of morbidity, in addition to mortality (see Section 4.2).

Life tables and life expectancy

Life tables are a type of *survival analysis*—a powerful means of summarizing the occurrence of mortality or other health events (e.g., complications, new cases of disease) in defined populations. Several variants exist, the main distinctions being the method of defining time intervals, and the requirement for the precise timing of the events (death, loss to follow-up, censoring) affecting each individual. The *product-limit* (Kaplan-Meier) approach (Selvin, 1991; 287 ff.) defines the end of a time interval as each time that an event occurs, and therefore does not have to deal with events during intervals. Because it requires precise follow-up information on each individual and (previously) a large amount of manual calculation, it has been used primarily in clinical situations with relatively small sample sizes. The *actuarial* (Cutler-Ederer) approach (Shyrock and Siegel, 1976: 251–4; Chiang, 1984:113–34) uses equal time intervals and makes assumptions enabling it to deal with events occurring during the intervals; usually this approach assumes that the events all occur at midpoints of the intervals. The actuarial approach can be used in both clinical situations (where follow-up information is available for each subject and there may be losses to follow-up) and demography (where data are available only for age-groups and it is assumed that there are no losses to follow-up).

The *demographic (population) life table* is a basic tool for policy epidemiology, the most common type being the *cross-sectional* or *period life table,* in which age-specific mortality rates for a specific year are used to estimate the lifetime experience of a hypothetical cohort of individuals born that year. Thus, it assumes that current mortality rates will continue throughout the lifetime of these individuals. Although this is obviously an incorrect assumption, it allows the calculation of *life expectancy*, a very useful summary measure of all age-specific mortality rates, which is not dependent upon any reference population and may therefore be compared across populations. A *cohort* or *generation life table* directly depicts the experience of a birth cohort across its entire life span, but the result is of only historical interest, since such a table cannot be completed until roughly a century after the birth of the cohort.

Complete or *unabridged life tables* provide entries for single years of age. The core of the calculation is the estimation of age-specific probabilities of death from age-specific mortality rates, the only data entering the life table. The usual approach reconstructs the cohort that gave rise to the mortality in a given year:

$$N = N_0 - (1 - f)d$$
$$N_0 = N + (1 - f)d$$

where d is the number of deaths, N_0 the size of a cohort at the beginning of the year, N the average (usually mid-year) population, and f the average proportion of a full year lived by each individual who dies during the year. The probability of death, q, is then

$$q = \frac{d}{N_0} = \frac{d}{N + (1 - f)d} = \frac{M}{1 + (1 - f)M}$$

where M is the mortality rate. Beyond age 4, it is safe to assume that $f = 0.5$, so the formula reduces to

$$q = \frac{d}{N + 0.5d} = \frac{M}{1 + \dfrac{M}{2}}$$

Figure 2-1 illustrates the basis of this conversion. For the first 5 years of life, more accurate fractions are 0.09, 0.43, 0.45, 0.47, and 0.49 years, respectively (Chiang, 1984:119), but some countries generate their own empirical data for survival at these early ages. Especially when the population is rather small, the single-year probabilities are often smoothed to remove irregularities. The demographic life table was developed long before modern epidemiology emerged, so its terminology and methods differ from current epidemiologic usage. Obviously, q is equivalent to cumulative mortality (CM) and M to mortality density (MD); the conversion formula presented above yields very similar results to the modern epidemiologic formula (CM $= 1 - e^{-MD \cdot t}$), when $t = 1$ year and the probability of death is low.

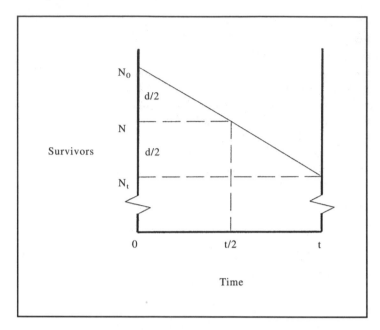

Figure 2-1. Basis of conversion from initial cohort to average population at risk. N_0 is the initial size of the cohort, N_t is its size at time t (normally 1 year), and N is its size at time $t/2$ (mid-year), which estimates the average population at risk. The deaths (d) are assumed to be spread equally over the year.

Once the age-specific probabilities of death have been calculated, construction of the life table is fairly straightforward. An initial birth cohort of 100,000 (l, the radix of the table) is assumed, the age-specific probabilities (q) are applied to the population at the beginning of each year to estimate the number of deaths during that year (d), and these deaths are subtracted from the population to indicate the number of persons alive at the beginning of the next year. Note that this value exactly equals the radix times the cumulative probability of not dying: $l_{x+1} = 100{,}000 \, \Pi \, (1 - q_x)$, as would be calculated in a clinical survival analysis (Selvin, 1991:281). But the life table goes further. The total number of years lived during each year (L) is calculated, using a value of 1 for those who survived the year and an average of 0.5 for those who died (for ages 0–4, the fractions presented in the previous paragraph are used). A different approach must be used for the highest age considered by the table, since this interval is open ended. It depends upon the fact that $d/L = M$, the population death rate, so that $L = d/M$ and therefore (since all the people arriving at this interval die) $L = l/M$. Alternatively, if the life table is extended to an advanced age, q may be simply set to 1 for the last row of the table. The years lived are then accumulated, beginning at the bottom of the table, to provide an estimate of the number of years yet to be lived (T) by people at each age. Dividing this number by the size of the cohort (l) at each age provides an estimate of the remaining life expectancy (e). In general, life expectancy drops with increasing age, but there are one or two exceptions: the first year of life and (in some populations) young men. Both of these ages are so hazardous that life expectancy actually increases for those who survive them. Also, in general, the sum of the current age and the remaining life expectancy increases with increasing age, as people have survived earlier hazards. It is possible to calculate the probability that a person of one age x will survive to another age y (l_y/l_x). Finally, the *stationary (life-table) population,* shown by the L column, shows what the age composition of the population would eventually become under the (artificial) conditions of a constant number of births and unchanging age-specific mortality rates, and the crude *life-table death rate* is l_0/T_0 or $1/e_0$. Table 2-1 illustrates the calculations with a Canadian life table from the early 1990s (adapted from Millar and David, 1995); although the values of L have been calculated as described above, the estimated life expectancies are virtually identical to those in the published table, which used a more complicated procedure.

Abridged life tables, based on 5-year age-groups, are often preferred for their brevity and because they are less vulnerable to the unstable rates arising from small populations. Several approximations exist to estimate the necessary probabilities from the 5-year death rates (Chiang, 1984:137–51; Shyrock and Siegel, 1976:254–7).

More advanced life tables. The *multiple-decrement (multiple-cause) life table* (Selvin, 1991:263–9) provides separate columns for deaths from various causes. For each age, the proportion of all deaths due to a specific cause (i.e., the proportionate mortality) can be multiplied times the number of life table deaths (column d) to estimate the deaths attributable to that cause. The total of these values across all ages, divided by 100,000, estimates the *lifetime probability of death from a specific cause,* in the presence of competing causes. Adjustment for competing risks (see below) allows the preparation of a *cause-elimination life table* (Peron and Strohmenger, 1985:175–81), which uses the net probabilities of death for all other causes after a specified cause has been eliminated, thus providing an estimate of the life expectancy under those conditions. Comparison with a conventional life table allows estimation of the *life expectancy lost* due to that cause and the gain that might be expected from its elimination (illustrated in Box 2–1). *Multistate life tables* incorporate the probability of developing reversible states like marriage or disability. Section 2.2 presents a way of incorporating *morbidity information* into a life table. Finally, *model life tables* (Coale and Demeny, 1966; United Nations, 1955) have been produced to represent the experience of countries that lack adequate demographic statistics to generate their own life tables; these were used in the World Bank's Global Burden of Disease project (Murray and Lopez, 1996a).

Table 2-1. Demographic Life Table: Canadian Females, 1990–92

Age (x)	Cohort Size (l_x)	Probability of Death (q_x)	No. of Deaths (d_x)	Proportion of Year Lived (f_x)	Years Lived in Interval (L_x)	Years Yet to Live (T_x)	Life Expectancy (e)
	$l_{x-1} - d_{x-1}$	$M_x/(1+(1-f_x)M_x)$	$l_x q_x$	Chiang (1984)	$l_x - (1-f_x)d_x$	$T_{x+1} + L_x$	T_x/l_x
Source							
0	100,000	0.00577	577	0.09	99,475	8,089,540	80.90
1	99,423	0.00045	45	0.43	99,397	7,990,065	80.36
2	99,378	0.00030	30	0.45	99,362	7,890,667	79.40
3	99,348	0.00024	24	0.47	99,336	7,791,305	78.42
4	98,325	0.00018	18	0.49	99,315	7,691,969	77.44
5	99,307	0.00014	14	0.50	99,300	7,592,654	76.46
6	99,293	0.00013	13	0.50	99,286	7,493,354	75.47
104	468	0.42582	199	0.50	368	648	1.39
105	269	0.45725	123	0.50	207	280	1.04
106	146	1.00000	146	0.50	73	73	0.50

M_x, age-specific death rates observed in the population.
Source: Data from Millar and David (1995: 4–5).

Box 2-1 Effect of eliminating a disease group on life expectancy

Nusselder et al. (1996) studied the effects of eliminating various diseases on the life expectancy of the Dutch population. A first step was to calculate net probabilities of death from all other causes, after elimination of these diseases. Although these calculations were done on an age-specific basis, they can be demonstrated using the published crude rates; for these low probabilities, it is safe to assume that the probability of death in 1 year equals the death rate. Selected results were as follows:

Disease Group Considered	Crude Probability	Net Probability after Eliminating i (q_i)	
		Exponential	Intuitive
All causes (q)	0.0445		
Arthritis/back complaints (Q_i)	0.0004		
All other causes	0.0441	0.044109	0.044109
Cancer (Q_i)	0.0093		
All other causes	0.0352	0.035367	0.035364

The net probabilities of death from all other causes were used to construct two cause-deleted life tables, and the resulting life expectancies compared with that calculated in a standard life table. The findings for life expectancy of women at age 15 years were as follows:

Disease Group to be Eliminated	Before Elimination (years)	After Elimination (years)	Effect of Elimination (years)
Arthritis/back complaints	65.6	65.7	+0.1
Cancer	65.6	68.9	+3.3

Thus, elimination of arthritis and back complaints (generally nonfatal diseases) would produce only minimal change in life expectancy, whereas elimination of cancer (a relatively fatal disease) would lead to a fairly substantial increase.

Competing risks

Individuals are subject to concurrently operating forces of mortality from many diseases. If mortality from one condition drops, then individuals will be at risk of death from other conditions for more person-years, and the mortality rate from those other causes will increase slightly. Adjustment for these competing risks distinguishes between the *crude proba-*

bility, Q_i of death from cause *i* (as observed in the presence of other causes of death, and obtained from ordinary cause-specific death rates) and the *net probability, q_i* of death from the cause (the probability when all other causes have been eliminated). The *partial crude probability* of death from a cause when some but not all other causes have been eliminated is also sometimes defined. The most useful application is the calculation of $q_{\cdot i}$, the net probability of death from all remaining causes after cause *i* has been eliminated, which is given by Chiang (1991) as

$$q_{\cdot i} = 1 - p \ \frac{q - Q_i}{q} = 1 - (1 - q) \ \frac{q - Q_i}{q}$$

where *q* is the probability of dying from any cause and *p* is the probability of surviving the interval (in the presence of all causes of death), so that *p* + *q* = 1. The exponent is a proportional mortality and reflects Chiang's "proportionality assumption," i.e., that a cause accounts for a constant proportion of the force of mortality from all causes during a given time interval. Approaching the problem from a more intuitive angle yields another estimate (Selvin, 1991:274–5):

$$q_{\cdot i} = \frac{d - d_i}{1 - 0.5 d_i}$$

where *d* is the total number of deaths, d_i is the deaths from the cause to be eliminated, and *l* is the number of persons at risk.

Box 2-1 illustrates the results of a cause-elimination life table prepared using $q_{\cdot i}$, the net probability of death from all other causes, for the *q* column.

Fatality

Fatality (often called case-fatality) refers to the occurrence of death among persons suffering from a disease, and is important for what it says about the severity of the disease and the effects of health care. Unfortunately, its users often fail to specify either the causes of death included or the type of indicator used. On the first point, it is often not specified whether case-fatality refers to deaths from the disease of interest (as derived from mortality statistics) or to deaths from all causes among persons with the disease. The latter is often more appropriate when dealing with chronic diseases or with the elderly, but cannot be calculated from population data unless the "other significant conditions contributing to the . . . death" on the death certificate is coded, which is not usually the case. On the second point, fatality is almost always called a rate (density), but is more often actually a probability (cumulative fatality). In a clinical setting, the dates of disease onset and death are usually known for individuals, so both the fatality density and the cumulative fatality can be calculated directly. In a population setting no such individualized information is available, but fatality can sometimes be estimated indirectly, in the form of a lifetime risk (cumulative incidence measure), from the relation:

$$\text{Lifetime Cumulative Fatality} \approx \frac{\text{Mortality Density}}{\text{Incidence Density}}$$

For this relation to hold, the condition must be rare and steady-state conditions must prevail. Further details are provided by Kleinbaum et al. (1982:126).

2.2 Composite Indicators of Health

For many purposes it is desirable to have a single summary indicator of the health status of a population (Patrick and Bergner, 1990). This might be used to monitor changes in health status, identify populations with particularly bad health, evaluate health programs, or model the impact of a policy on population health. Various formulations exist, all of which are dependent on weighting the morbid states by severity. Development of these measures has been multidisciplinary, involving economists, demographers and clinical epidemiologists.

Quality-Adjusted Life Years, Disability-Adjusted Life Years, and Related Measures

The number of years that an individual or population spends in each health state can be multiplied by the weight for that state to convert it to *quality-adjusted life years* (QALYs). The investigator wishing to use these indicators will need a health measurement scale that yields a single score. Generalized scales like the EuroQol Quality of Life Scale (EuroQol Group, 1990) or the McMaster Health Utility Index (Boyle et al., 1995) provide such a score, but for some purposes it may be better to develop a scale specific to the situation being studied. The choice involves the usual trade-off between internal and external validity. In developing such a scale, discrete categories of health are defined, and each is assigned a weight ranging from 0 (for death, acknowledging that some states of "health" may be worse than death) to 1.0 (for perfect health). These weights are expressions of people's *preferences* for various states, based on the *utilities* (values) of the states to them. The preferences may be generated by methods ranging from the simple (visual analogue scale, "feeling thermometer") to the complex (time or person trade-offs, standard gamble) (Torrance, 1986). There is an extensive literature on whose preferences should be measured (perhaps only those who have experienced a state can evaluate it), and ample room for undervaluing certain population groups, e.g., elders. Indeed, the use of QALYs may set various age-groups in opposition to one another, and thus be socially divisive. At present the QALY is somewhat ill-defined, as it is calculated differently by different investigators. The World Bank project on global health (Murray, 1994) introduced the *disability-adjusted life year* (DALY), which is similar in concept to the QALY but differs in several details: (1) it is always calculated in the same way, so a DALY is a standardized QALY; (2) the direction of the scaling is reversed: 0 represents perfect health and 1 represents death; (3) there is discounting of future benefits at 3%; and (4) age weights are used, with larger weights being assigned to life years in the socially valuable middle ages than to life years in childhood or old age. *Healthy years equivalents* (HYEs) have been proposed as an alternative to QALYs (Mehrez and Gafni, 1989) on the grounds that QALYs only partly reflect an individual's true preferences. Any of these measures can be used in demographic (see next section), epidemiologic, or economic analyses.

Healthy Life Expectancy

Calculation of *healthy life expectancy* (health expectancy, life expectancy in good health) introduces morbidity into a life table. The usual approach, suggested by Sullivan (1971), breaks down life expectancy into several disability categories. The years lived by the cohort at each age (L_x) are allocated to various health states, based on cross-sectional population data, yielding several L_x columns and life expectancies, one for each level of health. Tables 2-2 and 2-3 provide an example, using data drawn from the 1978 Canadian abridged life table and the Canadian Health Survey of 1978, and show that the average Canadian could expect to live 70.8 years, of which 59.2 would be free of significant disability (healthy life expectancy), 10.8 years would be disabled but in the community, and 0.8 years would be in institutional care (Wilkins and Adams, 1983). The Remaining Years Lived column in Table 2-3 is needed to provide the correct denominator for the remaining categories, as the Canada Health Survey included only the noninstitutionalized population.

Box 2-2 combines the concepts of disability-free life expectancy and cause-elimination life tables to show the effect of eliminating a disease on healthy life expectancy.

Health-Adjusted Life Expectancy

Alternatively, a single L_x column can contain the total QALYs lived in each interval, so that life expectancy (LE) becomes *quality-adjusted life expectancy* (QALE), increasingly called *health-adjusted life expectancy* (HALE).

Table 2-2. Calculation of Health Expectancy, Canadian Males, 1978: Institutionalization

Age (x)	Survivors (l_x)	Years Lived (L_x)	Years Yet To Live (T_x)	LE (e_x)	Proportion in Institutions (PI_x)	Years Lived in Institutions (LL_x)	Years Yet To Live in Institutions (TI_x)	LE in Institutions (eI_x)
Source	Life table	Life table	Sum from bottom	T_x/l_x	Institutional reports	$L_x \times PI_x$	Sum from bottom	TI_x/l_x
0	100,000	1,475,419	7,080,818	70.8	0.00204	3,008	75,703	0.8
15	98,004	972,823	5,605,399	57.2	0.00292	2,838	72,695	0.7
25	96,408	1,896,306	4,632,576	48.1	0.00274	5,196	69,857	0.7
45	92,509	1,699,064	2,736,270	29.6	0.00592	10,050	64,661	0.7
65+	72,274	1,037,206	1,037,206	14.4	0.05265	54,611	54,611	0.8

LE, life expectancy.

Source: Adapted from Wilkins and Adams (1983:71), with permission.

Table 2-3. Calculation of Health Expectancy, Canadian Males, 1978: Noninstitutionalized Disability

Age (x)	Remaining Years Lived (TR_x)	Proportion Disabled (PD_x)	Years Lived Disabled (LD_x)	Years Yet To Live Disabled (TD_x)	LE Disabled (eD_x)	Years Lived in Health (LH_x)	Years Yet To Live in Health (TH_x)	LE in Health (eH_x)
Source	$L_x - LI_x$	Health survey	$TR_x \times PD_x$	Sum from bottom	TD_x/l_x	$TR_x \times (1 - PD_x)$	Sum from bottom	TH_x/l_x
0	1,472,411	0.0543	79,981	1,081,271	10.8	1,392,430	5,923,844	59.2
15	969,985	0.0656	63,641	1,001,290	10.2	906,344	4,531,414	46.2
25	1,891,110	0.0891	168,403	937,649	9.7	1,722,707	3,625,070	37.6
45	1,689,014	0.22837	385,720	769,246	8.3	1,303,294	1,902,363	20.6
65+	982,595	0.39032	383,526	383,526	5.3	599,069	599,069	8.3

LE, life expectancy.

Source: Adapted from Wilkins and Adams (1983:79), with permission.

Box 2-2 Effect of eliminating a disease group on disability-free life expectancy

Nusselder et al. (see Box 2-1) extended their study to include disability-free life expectancy, using methods similar to those described in the text. Selected results for women aged 15 years were as follows:

Disease Group	Life expectancy (net change)			
	Total (years)	Disability-Free (years)	With Disability (years)	% with Disability
Baseline	65.6	45.6	20.0	30.5
After eliminating:				
Arthritis/back complaints	65.7 (+0.1)	48.4 (+2.8)	17.3 (–2.7)	26.3 (–4.2)
Cancer	68.9 (+3.3)	46.7 (+1.1)	22.2 (+2.2)	32.2 (+1.7)

Thus, elimination of arthritis and back complaints (disabling but non-fatal diseases) would result in compression of morbidity (absolute 2.7 years, relative 4.2 percentage points), whereas elimination of cancer (an often fatal disease that kills relatively quickly) would lead to expansion of morbidity (absolute 2.2 years, relative 1.7 percentage points).

Table 2-4 provides an illustration using the data from Tables 2-2 and 2-3. For this analysis, life in an institution was arbitrarily assigned a utility of 0.40 and life outside an institution but with a disability a utility of 0.57 (the weighted average of several categories of disability that were considered in Wilkins and Adams, 1983). The 70.8 total years of life expectancy turn out to be equivalent to 65.7 quality-adjusted (fully healthy) years.

The various indicators of life and health expectancy are related, as illustrated in Figure 2-2. Here we see that

1. (total) LE implicitly assigns a weight of 1 to all life years, regardless of health (70.8 years in Table 2-2);
2. HALE assigns weights to each state according to disability level or quality of life (65.7 years in Table 2-4);
3. Health expectancy (HE) or life expectancy in good health implicitly assigns a weight of 0 to all states of less than perfect health (59.2 years in Table 2-3).

Table 2-4. Calculation of Health-Adjusted Life Expectancy, Canadian Males, 1978

Age (x)	Survivors (l$_x$)	Years Lived in Institutions (LI$_x$)	Adjusted Years in Institutions (ALI$_x$)	Years Lived Disabled (LD$_x$)	Adjusted Years Disabled (ALD$_x$)	Years Lived in Health (LH$_x$)	Total Adjusted Years (AL$_x$)	Adjusted Years Yet To Live (AT$_x$)	Health Adjusted LE (HALE$_x$)
Source	Table 2-2	Table 2-2	LI$_x$*0.40	Table 2-3	LD$_x$*0.57	Table 2-3	ALI$_x$ + ALD$_x$ + LH$_x$	Sum from bottom	AT$_x$/l$_x$
0	100,000	3,008	1,203	79,981	45,589	1,392,430	1,439,222	6,570,448	65.7
15	98,004	2,838	1,135	63,641	36,275	906,344	943,754	5,131,226	52.4
25	96,408	5,196	2,078	168,403	95,990	1,722,707	1,820,775	4,187,472	43.4
45	92,509	10,050	4,020	385,720	219,860	1,303,294	1,527,174	2,366,697	25.6
65+	72,274	54,611	21,844	383,526	218,610	599,069	839,523	839,523	11.6

LE, life expectancy.
Source: Adapted from Wilkins and Adams (1983:79), with permission.

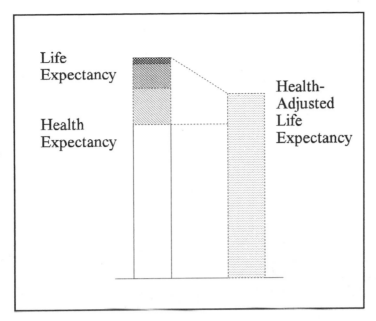

Figure 2-2. Relations among life expectancy (*LE*), health expectancy (*HE*), health-adjusted life expectancy (*HALE*). The shaded areas in the left bar indicate varying degrees of illness or disability. The right bar is a weighted average of all the components of the left bar, and is necessarily greater than health expectancy but less than life expectancy.

2.3 Epidemiologic Indicators of Effect

Indicators of Association

These indicators take the form of ratio and difference indicators, known generically as *relative risk* (RR) and *attributable risk* (AR). Neither term is very precise, since relative risk can take the form of a risk ratio (cumulative incidence ratio [CIR]), rate ratio (incidence density ratio [IDR]) or odds ratio (OR), and attributable risk can be either a risk difference (cumulative incidence difference [CID]) or a rate difference (incidence density difference [IDD]). Two topics require discussion here: generalizability and choice of indicator.

Generalizability of published research results
For policy purposes, it is often necessary to draw data from several studies or other sources. Several questions arise regarding the interpretation of published indicators of association and the ability to combine them. The relevant literature refers to RRs, but the points apply equally to ARs.

Which relative risk? The various types of RR are sometimes confused, most commonly by using the odds ratio to estimate the rate ratio when this is not justified. The odds ratio has different interpretations under different case–referent study designs (Pearce, 1993), estimating the risk ratio in case-base and case–cohort studies, the rate ratio in prospective case-control studies with density sampling and nested case–control studies, and the population odds ratio in retrospective case–control studies. Rate ratio and risk ratio may also be confused, as when an "RR of 3" is cited without specifying which variant is being used.

Time issues. In the case of risks, the duration of observation may be different from the period of exposure of interest to a policymaker (requiring adjustment, which may or not be methodologically valid), or may not be specified (making the statistic uninterpretable). In the case of rates, all person-years may have been considered identical, despite the possibility that period or cohort effects may be present (stratification is desirable).

Assumptions of uniformity. It is common to assume that a given RR applies to all age- and sex-groups, when in fact, RRs often appear to decline with advancing age. It is uncertain whether this represents a true diminution in effect, or is an artefact due to differential survival (van de Mheen and Gunning-Schepers, 1996).

Crude versus specific versus adjusted relative risks. For most purposes, RRs should be adjusted for confounders. But published RRs may not have been adjusted adequately for certain covariates, and cannot have been adjusted for covariates that were not measured. The published RR is crude (unadjusted) with respect to such covariates, and may be confounded by them. The crude RR equals the adjusted RR only when the data fit the multiplicative model, and the crude AR equals the adjusted AR only when the data fit the additive model, but these facts are of limited value since in cases where one knows the causal model, one probably has appropriately adjusted indicators available.

Ratio or difference indicators?

For policy purposes, ratio indicators often miss the mark, as a large ratio can be associated with a very low baseline risk, so the risk among the exposed may still be low in absolute terms. Policymakers (and the public) should be more interested in absolute indicators (Rose, 1992:39). Attributable risk, a difference indicator, measures the absolute burden of disease associated with an exposure, and should only be used when an association is believed to be causal. In principle, two variants exist:

Exposed Attributable Risk

$$EAR = I_E - I_U = (RR - 1) I_U$$

Population Attributable Risk

$$PAR = I_T - I_U = pI_E + (1 - p) I_U - I_U$$
$$= p (RR - 1) I_U \text{ (dichotomous)}$$
$$PAR = (\Sigma pI) - I_U$$
$$= (\Sigma pRR - 1) I_U \text{ (polychotomous)}$$

where I_E, I_U, and I_T are incidence (CI or ID) in the exposed and unexposed groups and overall, and p is the prevalence of exposure.

The *exposed attributable risk* (EAR) contrasts the exposed group to the unexposed group and thus measures the risk in the exposed group that is attributable to the exposure. In practice, this statistic is simply called *attributable risk*. The *population attributable risk* (PAR) is a less common statistic that compares the overall incidence in the population to the incidence in unexposed persons (note that the term is often imprecisely used to refer to a fraction, rather than a difference). The PAR is useful in that it estimates the absolute amount of disease in the whole population that can be attributed to an exposure such as smoking or poverty, but appears mainly as a component of the population attributable fraction (see below).

Since ARs require an estimate of incidence, they are not available from case–control studies, although the OR can be used to estimate the *excess relative risk*, RR–1, which is sometimes useful. If information is available from some other source on the prevalence of exposure (p) and on the overall incidence of the disease in the population (I_T), then the incidence in the exposed and unexposed groups (I_E and I_U) can be estimated from the relationship:

$$I_T = pI_E + (1 - p)\, I_U = [1 + p(RR - 1)]\, I_U \text{ (dichotomous)}$$
$$I_T = \Sigma pI = (\Sigma pRR)\, I_U \text{ (polychotomous)}$$

solving first for I_U, then for I_E. The attributable risks can then estimated.

Clinical epidemiologists recognize the importance of absolute risk when they calculate *absolute risk reduction* (ARR) and *number needed to treat,* (NNT) (Laupacis et al., 1988; Sackett et al., 1991:205). Since clinical interventions (generally) reduce risk, the calculations are the opposite of attributable risk:

$$ARR = CI_U - CI_E = - CID$$

The NNT estimates the number of individuals whose exposure to a hazard would need to be eliminated to prevent one case of a disease; thus the NNT assists in assessing clinical significance:

$$NTT = \frac{1}{ARR} = \frac{1}{|CID|}$$

Indicators of Potential Impact

These indicators are the most important ones for policy purposes, because they illustrate the impact of an exposure or a program on a population group. Unfortunately, they labor under a welter of names, shown in Table 2-5. The basic distinctions are whether the exposure is hazardous or protective, and whether the target group is the exposed or the whole

Table 2-5. Indicators of Potential Impact: Terminology

Exposure	Exposed Population	Whole Population
Hazardous	Exposed attributable fraction	Population attributable fraction
	Exposed etiologic fraction	Population etiologic fraction
	Relative attributable risk	Population attributable risk proportion
	Attributable risk %	Population attributable risk %
Protective	Exposed prevented fraction	Population prevented fraction
	Exposed prevented fraction	Population prevented fraction
	Relative risk reduction	
	Vaccine efficacy	Vaccine effectiveness
Either	Impact fraction	Impact fraction

population. Because these statistics are based on ARs, they should only be used when it has been concluded that an association is causal.

Attributable fractions
Attributable fractions are used for hazardous exposures (RR > 1). The basic concept behind attributable fractions is illustrated by the simple diagrams in Figure 2-3 for both the exposed and the total populations. In the following section, the right-hand column builds on the formula for I_T from the previous section.

Exposed Attributable Fraction

$$EAF = \frac{I_E - I_U}{I_E}$$

$$= \frac{RR-1}{RR} = 1 - \frac{1}{RR}$$

Population Attributable Fraction

$$PAF = \frac{I_T - I_U}{I_T} = \frac{pI_E + (1-p) I_U - I_U}{pI_E + (1-p) I_U}$$

$$= \frac{p(RR-1)}{1 + p(RR-1)} \text{ (dichotomous)}$$

$$PAF = \frac{(\Sigma pRR) - 1}{\Sigma pRR}$$

$$= 1 - \frac{1}{\Sigma pRR} \text{ (polychotomous)}$$

The attributable fractions indicate the proportion of an outcome that can be attributed to a certain risk factor, and thus the proportion that can potentially be prevented by modifying the risk factor. The PAF is the most important epidemiologic indicator for policy purposes, because it illustrates the impact of a hazardous exposure on a whole population, e.g., the proportion of all deaths due to cigarette smoking. It is also the basis of much disease modeling (see Section 6.2). Box 2-3 provides a simple example.

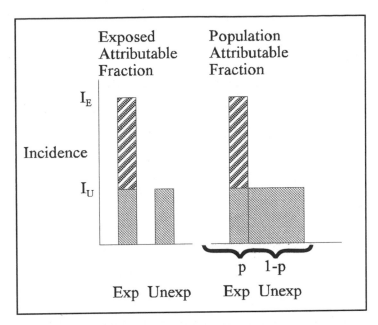

Figure 2-3. Attributable fractions. I_E and I_U are the incidence in the exposed and unexposed groups, p is the proportion of the population that is exposed, and $1-p$ the proportion not exposed. The hatched area represents cases that are attributable to the exposure (attributable risk, AR) and that would not have occurred in the absence of the exposure. It is assumed that in the absence of this hazardous exposure, the incidence would be I_U in the whole population.

Box 2-3. Attributable fractions

Consider a population with the following exposures to a hazardous agent, with the indicated risks for developing a certain disease:

Exposure Level	Prevalence	Incidence	RR	pRR
Not exposed	0.60	0.030/year	1.0	0.60
Exposed	0.40	0.060/year	2.0	0.80
TOTAL	1.00	0.042/year	(1.4)	1.40

Exposed attributable risk (EAR) = 0.060 – 0.030 = 0.030/year. Among exposed individuals, 30 cases per 1000 person-years of exposure can be attributed to the exposure.

Exposed attributable fraction (EAF) = 0.030/0.060 or 1 – (1/2) = 0.50 or 50%. Half of all the cases in the exposed group can be attributed to their exposure.

Population attributable risk (PAR) = 0.042 – 0.030 = 0.012/year. In the entire population, 12 cases per 1000 person-years of observation can be attributed to this exposure.

Population attributable fraction (PAF) = 0.012/0.042 or (0.40 × 1.0)/ (1 + 0.40 × 1.0) = 0.29; i.e., 29% of all the cases in the population can be attributed to this exposure.

Prevented fractions

Miettinen (1974) suggested the use of the *prevented (preventive) fraction* for protective exposures (RR < 1). The reference point here is the incidence of disease that would occur if none of the population was exposed, and the fraction indicates the proportion of that (maximum) amount of disease that has (already) been prevented by exposure or intervention (Fig. 2-4).

Exposed Prevented Fraction

$$\text{EPF} = \frac{I_U - I_E}{I_U}$$

$$= 1 - \text{RR}$$

Population Prevented Fraction

$$\text{PPF} = \frac{I_U - I_T}{I_U} = \frac{I_U - pI_E - (1-p)I_U}{I_U}$$

$$= p(1 - \text{RR}) \text{ (dichotomous)}$$

$$\text{PPF} = \frac{I_U - \Sigma pI_U}{I_U}$$

$$= 1 - \Sigma p\text{RR} \text{ (polychotomous)}$$

Note that the exposed prevented fraction is identical to the *relative risk reduction* (RRR) used in clinical epidemiology (Sackett et al., 1991:203) and

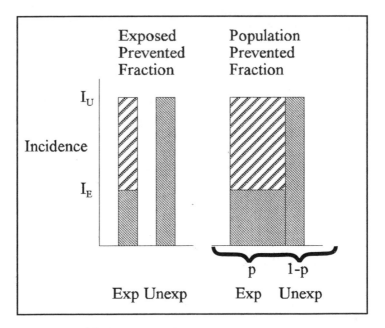

Figure 2-4. Prevented fractions. I_E and I_U are the incidence in the exposed and un-exposed groups, p is the proportion of the population that is exposed, and $1-p$ the proportion not exposed. The hatched area represents cases that have not occurred, having been prevented by the exposure, but that would have occurred in the absence of the exposure. It is assumed that in the absence of this protective exposure, the incidence would be I_U in the whole population.

to the *vaccine efficacy* used in communicable disease epidemiology (usually calculated as $1 - AR_V/AR_U$, where AR is the attack rate, or the cumulative incidence, in the vaccinated and unvaccinated groups). Haber et al., (1995) have suggested the use of *vaccine effectiveness*, which is analogous to the population prevented fraction $(1 - AR_T/AR_U)$. The analogy is not perfect because of the indirect effects of immunity (herd immunity): the attack rate in the absence of any immunization is not the same as the attack rate in the unimmunized in a population in which most people have been immunized.

The less commonly used *preventable fraction* is the proportion of disease, currently occurring in a population, that could be prevented if all currently unexposed persons were to receive a preventive intervention. The preventable fraction makes sense only at the population level:

$$\text{Preventable Fraction}$$

$$= \frac{I_T - I_E}{I_T}$$

$$= \frac{pI_E + (1-p)I_U - I_E}{pI_E + (1-p)I_U}$$

$$= \frac{(1-p)(1-RR)}{1 + p(1-RR)}$$

The fractions are related as follows:

$$I_T = I_U (1 - \text{Population Prevented Fraction})$$
$$I_E = I_T (1 - \text{Preventable Fraction})$$
$$\quad = I_U (1 - \text{Population Prevented Fraction})(1 - \text{Preventable Fraction})$$

See example in Box 2-4.

Impact fraction
The impact fraction extends the above concepts to situations where a hazardous exposure is not completely eliminated or where a preventive exposure does not achieve complete penetration:

$$\text{Impact Fraction} = \frac{I_1 - I_2}{I_1} = \frac{\Sigma(p_1 - p_2)\,RR}{\Sigma p_1 RR}$$

where the subscripts 1 and 2 refer to the higher and lower risk levels. This generalized version is the most useful member of the family (as will be illustrated in Section 6.2), and reduces to the other formulas when appropriate values of p are inserted.

Box 2-4. Prevented and preventable fractions

Consider a hypothetical epidemic in a population in which 40% of the people had been immunized, and in which the cumulative incidence of the disease was 10% in unimmunized persons and 2% in immunized persons:

State	Prevalence of State	Incidence of Disease	RR	pRR
Immunized (E)	0.4	0.020	0.2	0.008
Not immunized (U)	0.6	0.100	1.0	0.060
Total (T)	1.0	0.068	(0.68)	0.068

Exposed prevented fraction (EPF, equals vaccine efficacy) = $(0.10 - 0.02)/0.10 = 0.80$ or 80%. The immunization has reduced the incidence of the disease by 80% among immunized persons; the vaccine was 80% efficacious.

Population prevented fraction (PPF) = $(0.100 - 0.068)/0.100 = 0.32$ or 32%. The immunization program has reduced the incidence of the disease by 32% in the population as a whole; we might argue that the immunization program was 32% effective.

Preventable fraction = $(0.068 - 0.020)/0.068 = 0.71$ or 71%. This proportion of cases could have been prevented by increasing vaccine coverage from 40% to 100%.

Note that $(0.100)(1 - 0.32)(1 - 0.71) = 0.020$; the incidence in a completely unimmunized population multiplied by the proportion of cases remaining at the current immunization level multiplied by the proportion of cases remaining after immunization of the currently unimmunized persons equals the (irreducible) incidence in the immunized.

Behavior in the presence of multiple risk factors

Complications arise as soon as more than one risk factor is considered, since then there are possibilities for different causal models, for effect modification, and for confounding. These issues are of great importance in constructing disease models (see Section 6.2). How should one calculate the PAFs for the individual risk factors? Often the incidence is not available for each exposure level, so p and RR must be assembled from diverse sources. Ideally, the adjusted RR for each risk factor will be available, but the PAFs calculated from the adjusted RRs are correct only when the risk factors are not correlated. Even if they are correct, can the PAFs for two or more risk factors be added or multiplied to yield the combined effect of all the risk factors (the composite population attributable fraction)? Spasoff and McDowell (1987) present the situation in the context of health risk appraisal (Table 2-6; also see Section 4.3 on behavioral risk appraisal).

Table 2-6. Composite Attributable Fraction with Multiple Risk Factors

Causal Model	RFs Independent	RFs Correlated
Multiplicative	$1 - \Pi\{1 - PAF_i\}$	Not possible to combine
Additive	$\Sigma\, PAF_i$	$\Sigma\, PAF_i$
All other	Not possible to combine	Not possible to combine

A considerable literature exists on how to deal with these issues (Walter, 1983). The ideal approach is probably to consider each *combination* of exposures as a separate stratum, as if all were levels of exposure to a single risk factor. This composite variable is unaffected by effect modification or confounding, but one will rarely have the necessary data to construct it accurately. Failing that, it seems reasonable to calculate PAFs separately for each variable (using adjusted RRs wherever possible), to add or multiply them as indicated in Table 2-6, and then to perform do sensitivity analyses to estimate the amount of error that has been introduced. Van de Mheen and Gunning-Schepers (1997) show that assuming independence of risk factor prevalences does not introduce substantial errors into the final result of the public health model Prevent (see Box 6-6).

Summary

Policy epidemiology emphasizes different indicators from those most used in etiological research. Fertility rates reflect reproductive performance and combine with population composition to yield birth rates. Potential years of life lost (PYLL) is often a more useful statistic than the number of deaths; results depend on the definition of "normal" age of death. Demographic life tables have many uses beyond showing life expectancy. Adjusting for competing risks allows preparation of cause-deleted life tables, which can be compared to ordinary life tables to show the gain in life expectancy that can be expected from elimination of a disease. Quality-adjusted life years (QALYs) and similar measures combine data on mortality and morbidity. Introduction of morbidity information into a life table yields health expectancy (HE) and health-adjusted life expectancy (HALE). Relationships between incidence, prevalence, and fatality are complicated; the well-known equation that fatality equals mortality divided by incidence refers to lifetime cumulative fatality. Attributable risk indicates the absolute burden associated with an exposure, and is often more relevant than relative risk. But the impact fraction and its variants are the epidemiologic indicators most relevant to health policy. When more than one risk factor is involved, the effects of effect modification and confounding must be considered.

Key References

Chiang CL. *The Life Table and Its Applications.* Malabar, FL: Robert E Krieger, 1984.

Kleinbaum DG, Kupper LL, Morgenstern H. *Epidemiologic Research: Principles and Quantitative Methods.* Belmont, CA: Lifetime Learning Publications, 1982; Chapter 7.

Murray CJL. Quantifying the burden of disease: the technical basis for disability-adjusted life years. Bull World Health Organ 1994;72:429–445.

Peron Y, Strohmenger C. *Demographic and Health Indicators: Presentation and Interpretation.* Ottawa: Statistics Canada, 1985 (Catalogue Number 82-543E).

Wilkins R, Adams O. *Healthfulness of Life.* Montreal: Institute for Research on Public Policy, 1983.

3

Population Health Data

Evidence-based health policy requires evidence, and much of that evidence comes in the form of population health data: vital statistics, health surveys, disease registries, and administrative databases generated by hospital and medical care insurance programs. The available information is always imperfect and insufficient, but decisions are made anyway; the epidemiologist's job is to ensure that the information is as strong as possible. Skills in epidemiology, computing, information systems, and planning are prerequisites. But before we can deal with health data, we must think about the meaning of health.

3.1 Conceptualizing Health

The definition of health, the ostensible goal of the entire health system, remains elusive, as it is differently interpreted by professionals, the public, and different disciplines. Traditionally, health was equated with survival, or absence of death; in fact, mortality is still used as a measure of (the absence of) health. The next stage was to see health as the absence of disease; this definition is still the most widely used in practice. But nearly everyone agrees that health is more than the absence of disease, and many attempts have been made at a broader definition. The usual starting point is the World Health Organization (WHO, 1947:13) description that health is "a state of complete physical, mental and social well-being and not merely the absence of disease or infirmity," and the usual next steps are to despair of applying this definition to specific situations, and to dismiss it as utopian. The definition does emphasize, however, the multidimensionality of health and the existence of positive health, and it serves as an ideal. Other approaches are less ambitious, referring to absence of disease, disability, or handicap. A physiological approach would suggest "normal" function at the cellular level, but this begs the question of what is normal (Sackett et al., 1991:58–60). Social scientists have contributed heavily to more recent conceptualizations. The Ottawa Charter for Health Promotion (World Health Organization, 1986) states that "[t]o reach a state of complete physical, mental and social well-being, an individual or group must be able to identify and to realize aspirations, to satisfy needs, and to change or cope with the environment. Health is, therefore, seen as a resource for everyday life, not the objective of living. Health is a positive concept emphasizing social and personal resources, as well as physical capacities." Thus, it offers a meaning for well-being, refers to the health of populations, and lends an active perspective. The idea that health is a resource or means for living, not the purpose or end, is consistent with the call in the WHO's Health for All declaration for all people to attain a level of health "that will permit them to lead a socially and economically productive life" (World Health Organization, 1981a:11). This broad definition of health is reflected in WHO-EURO's aims (goals) for health (World Health Organization, 1985), which are summarized as:

- Ensuring equity in health (health for all);
- Adding life to years (improving quality of life);
- Adding health to life (reducing morbidity);
- Adding years to life (reducing mortality).

Positive health is particularly hard to define, as it is open ended and inherently subjective. But there are plenty of attempts, including those that emphasize

- Psychological factors, or the realization of higher needs, such as self-actualization (Maslow, 1968:25–6);
- Ecological factors, or the ability to adapt to the environment and resist threats to the integrity of the organism (Dubos, 1965);
- Robustness, in the form of physical and mental fitness;
- Future health, which is the state of having a favorable prognosis (low risks, due to healthful lifestyle).

There is general acceptance that health is multidimensional and that it is possible simultaneously to score high on some dimensions and low on others. Therefore, developing a single index of an individual's health status is difficult and possibly inappropriate (although frequently attempted). The earlier emphasis on survival persists in use of mortality (or its steady-state reciprocal, life expectancy) as an indicator of health. This can have some unfortunate effects, e.g., the application of heroic therapy to maintain life, regardless of its quality. It is now widely recognized that we must focus on the *quality of life,* which is seen as a component of health, or even as its definition. But this concept tends to include all aspects of life, making it impossible to measure and difficult to relate to health interventions. There has therefore emerged the concept of *health-related quality of life,* which aims to include only those aspects directly relevant to health and amenable to health interventions. As defined by Patrick and Erickson (1993:22), it is "the value assigned to duration of life as modified by impairments, functional states, perceptions, and social opportunities that are influenced by disease, injury, treatment or policy." They conceive it as having five components (1993:77): opportunity; health perceptions; functional status, including social, psychological, and physical function; impairment; and death and duration of life.

Self-rated health offers an integrated approach that incorporates an individual's own perceptions and priorities and correlates with more complex indices (Rowan, 1994) and future mortality (Idler and Benyamini, 1997).

Despite the interest in and acknowledgement of positive health, we most often adapt (consciously or unconsciously) a restricted definition, i.e., absence of disease or infirmity, and then measure deviations from that limited state. This book will follow that course, emphasizing measurement of the absence of health. This is somewhat defensible in that the highest priority should presumably be given to the most immediate health problems, with positive health assuming a lower priority (cf. Maslow's [1968] hierarchy of human needs).

3.2 Health Data, Health Information, and Health Intelligence

Health data refers to unprocessed numbers or observations, e.g., numbers of deaths. When these are analyzed they become *health information* (National Task Force on Health Information, 1991), e.g., mortality rates, presented in the form of tables and graphs. Information needs both a sender and a receiver to be useful, which emphasizes the necessary partnership between producer and user of the information. When the information has been interpreted and its implications drawn out, it constitutes *health intelligence*,[1] e.g., discussion of the reasons for the observed patterns and of possible interventions. Health intelligence is necessary for making informed decisions.

Unfortunately, available information is often not optimally used. We appear to have a great many health data, considerably less health information, and still less health intelligence, partly because it is often easier to collect more data than to analyze and interpret those that are already available (especially if they have been collected without sufficient consideration of their use). Timeliness is essential: old data may no longer be relevant or politically convincing. A recurring example concerns health human resources (formerly health manpower), where rapid changes in migration and practice patterns run well ahead of available data. In the case of cohort studies and randomized trials, delay may be largely unavoidable; 20 years of follow-up will generally take at least 20 years, but in the case of descriptive data on health status and health services, long delays are inexcusable.

Health information technology is burgeoning, but most developments

---

[1]This distinction is said to have been suggested by Gordon MacLachlan; the reference is unknown to the author.

continue to focus on the institutional sector and are not population based (Friede et al., 1995). The focus here is on population-based health data, which are necessary to inform health policy. Epidemiology can make a particular contribution to such data, including their conceptualization, access, manipulation, and interpretation. This chapter addresses population health data and their conversion to health information, while Chapter 4 begins the process of using the health information (with the help of policymakers) to create health intelligence.

The World Wide Web has revolutionized the access to population health data (Laporte, 1994). Agencies like the National Center for Health Statistics, the Agency for Health Care Policy and Research, and Statistics Canada have created web sites from which data can be downloaded directly, often free of charge. Data availability and quality vary from one jurisdiction to another, but one can make some general comments (Williams and Young, 1996).

Scope of Health Data

Identification of the data needed to measure health is greatly facilitated by use of a model of health and its determinants. Of the many that exist, the one emerging from the population health movement (Evans and Stoddart, 1994), presented in Figure 3-1, encompasses both determinants

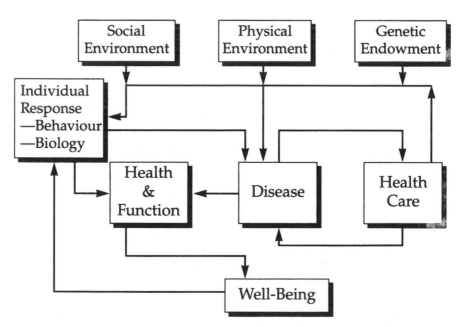

Figure 3-1. Conceptual framework of population health. [Reprinted with permission from: Evans, Robert G., Morris L. Barer, and Theodore R. Marmor (eds). Why Are Some People Healthy and Others Not? The Determinants of Health of Populations. (New York: Aldine de Gruyter) Copyright © 1994 Walter de Gruyter, Inc., New York.]

of health and the idea of positive health (well-being). The influence of Lalonde's (1974) health fields on this model is obvious. Krieger (1992) reminds us that the conceptual framework we use and the data we collect are strongly influenced by our values and by politics, and in turn strongly influence the uses of the data and the conclusions drawn from them.

Van der Maas et al. (1989:309) identify three types of public health information as relevant for policy: (1) health status, (2) health determinants, and (3) possibilities for intervention. To interpret them, and certainly to make projections into the future, it is also necessary to have data on the composition and characteristics of the population.

The Dutch health policy process (Ruwaard et al., 1994:30) uses the model presented in Figure 3-2 for indicators of *health status.*

The same process elaborates on Lalonde's (1974) health fields in classifying *health determinants* (here including interventions) as presented in Table 3-1.

Here we distinguish between the distribution of determinants and health services on the one hand, and the identification of determinants and the evaluation of health services on the other. The former come from population health data, the subject of Chapter 3 and most of Chapter 4. Identification of determinants and evaluation of health services are outside the scope of this book, but their interpretation is referred to at the end of Chapter 4 and in Chapter 5.

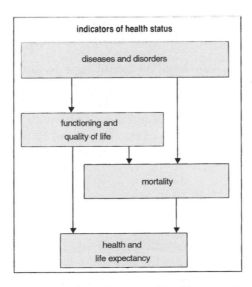

Figure 3-2. Conceptual model for indicators of health status. Integration of indicators increases toward the bottom of the schema. [From Ruwaard et al., 1992:30, with permission.]

Table 3-1. Health Determinants

Endogenous	Hereditary
	Acquired
Exogenous	Physical environment
	Lifestyle factors
	Social environment
Health care/prevention	Health care
	Somatic (physical)
	Mental
	Prevention
	Health protection
	Collective prevention
	Health promotion

Source: Adapted from Ruwaard et al. (1992:31), with permission.

Ruwaard et al. (1994:159–61) go on to distinguish five levels of health information, permitting increasingly valuable use of data:

- recording the situation at one moment in time for individual indicators;
- recording trends over time for individual variables;
- simultaneously recording a series of different variables;
- describing relationships among different indicators;
- making forecasts with the help of modeling. This highest level requires that data include determinants and indicators from all levels of the conceptual model, be nationally representative, be repeated regularly, and be linked to individuals as far as possible.

Most current data were found to constitute individual indicators at one moment in time, and it was rare to find data that showed trends over time or patterns over several indicators simultaneously, or that linked the layers of their conceptual model or made forecasts with the help of modeling. Similarly, a working group of the (Canadian) National Task Force on Health Information (1992) concluded that population health data should be "multi-multi-milo":

- *multi*variate (looking at various aspects of health and life);
- *multi*level (allowing analyses at the level of individuals, families, communities, etc.);
- *mi*crodata (oriented toward individuals);
- *lo*ngitudinal (following individuals over time).

But the Task Force acknowledged that few of the then available data met these criteria.

Fortunately, the suboptimal data that are available can support a great deal of health policy formulation and program planning. More realistic criteria for community health data (with common limitations identified) might be the following:

1. Consistent geographic reference, capable of aggregation to administrative boundaries. This is a frequent problem, since most denominator data are coded to the census and most numerator data are coded to postal codes; furthermore, administrative boundaries sometimes adjust to accommodate political and population changes, rendering longitudinal comparisons difficult.
2. Consistent coding of age-groups. This is rarely a problem, although privacy considerations may prevent use of the narrow age groupings that are often desirable for health planning.
3. Accuracy, including accurate recording of basic data, standardized coding schemes, and minimal coding errors. This pertains particularly to diagnoses on death certificates and physicians' claims and to many survey data.
4. Timeliness. Even when a census is conducted every 5 years, census data can be up to 7 years out of date, and mortality data are usually 2 or 3 years old.
5. Relevance to planning and evaluation needs. Many jurisdictions lack valid indicators of positive health and community health services, and some lack useful data on utilization of physicians' services.
6. Availability in machine-readable form. Such data are sometimes available only at higher cost than paper copies.
7. Accessibility. Privacy protection often prevents access to data for the small areas relevant to planning and evaluation, while the multiplicity of data holders and potential users makes for poor communication and much duplication of effort.
8. Availability at reasonable cost. The current tendency of governments to require their agencies to operate on a cost-recovery basis makes data relatively inaccessible to smaller and poorer users, including most potential researchers.

Individual and Aggregated Data

It is important to distinguish between *individual data* (microdata), in which the unit is the individual, and *aggregated data*, in which the unit of observation is the group.

Individual data (microdata)

One can envisage a "flat" file that lists all the individuals in a population on one dimension and all the variables on the other; the cells of the table contain the value of each variable for each individual. This simplest data format permits all sorts of detailed analysis, e.g., cross-tabulations and regressions. A file for a national population would contain millions of rows (records), one for each person, and one column (field) for each variable; it would thus be long and narrow.

Aggregated data

Microdata files are generally not available for the whole population, both because of their unwieldy size and to protect the confidentiality of individuals (given a microdata file of the entire census, a user might be able to identify the next-door neighbor and determine the income of that person). The data are therefore aggregated into summary tables, in which the unit of analysis is a group, e.g., the residents of a geographic area (province/state, municipality, census tract). There is then one row for each group, many fewer than in the microdata file. But it is no longer possible to assign only one column (field) to each variable, since the members of each group possess a variety of values. The table must therefore present a frequency distribution for each variable, using as many columns as there are categories (alternatively, only measures of central tendency could be recorded, but this loses information about the dispersion in the population). The overall file will be much shorter than the microdata file, but somewhat wider, as there is one field for each value of each variable. The data structures used by statistical agencies vary, and users of data from multiple sources (e.g., for rate calculations) must manipulate the data sets to create a common structure to combine them; this manipulation can be difficult, although various government and commercial agencies have developed computer programs to accomplish this automatically. Some files list totals as a separate category, providing (for example) three sexes, and introducing much duplication into the tables, since each individual appears not only in a cell but also in all of the relevant totals.

The essence of aggregated data is that individuals cannot be distinguished from other individuals with similar characteristics (of course, an individual might be identifiable if there are no other individuals with similar characteristics, which explains the data suppression rules that are built into such data files). Such files provide basic descriptive data and allow ecologic analyses (see Section 4.4). But the only cross-tabulations available are those already built into the file, in the form of composite variables. If the component variables have Li levels, then the composite variable will have $N = \Pi Li$ categories. These categories can be distributed between the rows and columns of the table in various ways, from N rows with one column to one row with N columns. Any of the formats can be converted into any of the other formats, although not necessarily easily. Working with such a file is quite different from working with microdata. For example, given microdata including age and sex, a user could generate a cross-tabulation of those variables. But given aggregate data offering separate breakdowns by age and by sex, it is impossible to fill in the cells of a table of age by sex; a prepared age-by-sex table must be obtained. Furthermore, such files cannot be linked to other data files on an individual basis.

Administrative versus Specially Collected Data

The term *administrative data* is used here to refer to data collected, usually by government, for some administrative purpose (e.g., keeping track of the population eligible for certain benefits, paying doctors or hospitals), but not primarily for research or surveillance purposes (Kuller, 1995). Such data have obvious advantages over specially collected data for monitoring health: (1) relative cheapness, if costs can be shared across several uses; (2) large sample size, usually covering the entire population; and (3) relative freedom from bias, since the data are collected blindly, without any hypothesis in mind and without any axes to grind on behalf of specific populations. The disadvantages may also be considerable: (1) the data were collected for a purpose other than measuring health status and will rarely be ideal for the latter purpose; (2) the secondary uses of the data may be relatively low priority for their custodians, resulting in limited access or long delays; and (3) privacy considerations may severely limit secondary uses of the data. Obviously, the best situation is one in which the various potential users of the data can agree in advance on specifications and can obtain the necessary consents.

Survey Data

Health surveys (Cartwright, 1983; Abramson, 1984) are useful for needs assessments and for goal and priority setting. Repeat surveys can assist in evaluating policies and programs by determining whether progress is being made in addressing health problems, and longitudinal (panel) surveys involving repeated interviews of the same individuals can even measure incidence. Surveys are relatively expensive (although use of the telephone can reduce costs), and local agencies often lack the resources and expertise to do an excellent job of conducting one. Furthermore, if their methods are not identical to those of other jurisdictions, the results of the various investigations will not be comparable. There are therefore real advantages to using national survey data: lower costs, probably better quality, and definitely higher comparability. Even if a local area does its own surveys, it should borrow methods from national or provincial surveys and compare its results to theirs.

National health surveys occupy a middle ground between specially collected and administrative data in that they are conducted to support health planning and policy, but not necessarily for the purposes of a particular policymaker (although an important policymaker may be able to influence the design and content of the survey and buy extra sample size). In addition to interviews and/or self-completed questionnaires, a few surveys include physical and laboratory examinations. Missing data are often imputed by inserting the values for similar individuals. The microdata are usually available on tape, permitting users to conduct their own analyses. A local agency can select data from its "own" respondents, make direct estimates of the prevalence of selected health problems or risk factors in its own district (if sample size is adequate), and compare them to the national average. But the sample size drawn from a particular area will often be quite small—perhaps enough to yield stable univariate estimates, but not enough to support many breakdowns by age, sex, or small area. For example, the Ontario Health Survey was the largest health survey ever conducted in Canada, with roughly 50,000 respondents, but local public health units were disappointed at the limited analyses permitted by the sample size of 1100 from each such unit. Sample size will almost never be adequate to define specific subpopulations with special health needs, but small group estimation techniques may circumvent some of these problems (see Section 4.1).

The sample design of major health surveys is usually complex, involving several stages (Korn and Graubard, 1991). The result is that individuals may have unequal probabilities of being selected into the sample, and may exhibit clustering.

Data are usually weighted to compensate for variations in sampling fractions and make the sample representative of the target population. The weights represent the number of individuals in the population that each sampled individual represents. When multiplied by the counts in each cell of a table, they inflate the results to depict the entire population, resulting in a correct point estimate. Although proper use of weights deals adequately with differences in sampling fractions, it cannot eliminate non-response bias. For example, many recent surveys have used telephone interviews with sampling by random digit dialing, and thus are subject to bias from the small proportion of the population without telephones and the larger proportion that is rarely home or will not answer calls from strangers (response rates have plummeted recently, especially in urban areas, often to below 40%). The weighting also increases the standard errors of the estimates, often substantially.

Multistage sampling involves the selection of clusters of individuals who resemble one another more than they resemble members of other clusters. This tendency is reflected in the *intraclass correlation coefficient*, δ (Moser and Kalton, 1971:104–6). Provided that correct weights are used to reflect differing probabilities of selection, the point estimates from such a study are usually correct, but their standard errors will be underestimated unless the clustering is taken into account, through using either the *design effect* (deff) or specialized software like SUDAAN (Research Triangle Institute, PO Box 12194, Research Triangle Park, NC 27709-2194). The design effect is a function of the sample design:

$$\text{Design Effect (deff)} = \frac{\text{Var}_{\text{cluster}}}{\text{Var}_{\text{srs}}} = \sqrt{1 + \delta (n - 1)}$$

where $\text{Var}_{\text{cluster}}$ is the correct variance, allowing for the clustering, Var_{srs} is the variance calculated as though the survey had used simple random sampling, and n is the size of each cluster. Obviously, deff is 1 when either $\delta = 0$ (no intraclass correlation) or $n = 1$ (no cluster sampling). Calculation of the "correct" estimates of variance is complicated, so publications often include the design effect for each key variable, to be multiplied by the variance based on the assumption of simple random sampling; sometimes deft is provided, which is the ratio of the corresponding standard errors (thus the square root of deff). Alternatively, a table or graph may be provided that allows one to estimate the standard error of a given statistic, based on the value of the statistic and the number of observations that produced it. These approaches are usually adequate for descriptive studies, but for analytic studies (those examining the relationship between variables), the use of specialized software is usually indicated. Some data agencies refuse to release cluster information, and thereby preclude use of such software.

Measurement error is another affliction of survey results. Rogan and Gladen (1978) argued that the results from prevalence surveys should be adjusted for less than perfect sensitivity and specificity of the research instrument. It can be easily be shown that

$$\text{Adjusted Prevalence} = \frac{\text{Apparent Prevalence} + \text{Specificity} - 1}{\text{Sensitivity} + \text{Specificity} - 1}$$

Although this practice seems entirely logical, it is almost never done.

Record Linkage

Record linkage refers to the drawing together of information on the same individual(s) from different places in the same data file or from two or more data files (Newcombe, 1988). Although this has long been done manually, its real power was unleashed when methods were developed for doing it electronically. Two major approaches exist: the *deterministic* approach, which looks for exact matches, generally requires that a unique identification number for each individual appear on all the files, and results in yes–no decisions, and the *probabilistic* approach, which uses a variety of types of information, such as place and date of birth and mother's maiden name, to determine the probability that two records apply to the same individual. Given the resistance of many societies to unique identifying numbers and the ease with which such numbers can be incorrectly recorded when they do exist, probabilistic linkage seems to be the more promising method. Working with all possible pairs of records, this essentially Bayesian approach begins with an a priori estimate of the odds that each pair of records relates to the same person, calculates the likelihood ratio that identical values for each of the variables available for the linkage process indicate a true match, chains the likelihood ratios together to produce a composite likelihood ratio, and uses this to calculate the revised odds that the two records relate to the same person. The likelihood ratios are based on the principle that identical uncommon values provide stronger evidence for a linkage than identical common values. Record linkage has become a powerful tool for epidemiology, both for etiological research, e.g., linking files with exposure and files with outcome information, and policy research, e.g., identifying multiple admissions of the same individual, tracking the total utilization by an individual, or making estimates of the incidence of non-notifiable disease (Nova Scotia–Saskatchewan Cardiovascular Disease Epidemiology Group, 1989; McLean et al., 1994). Once a highly specialized activity requiring special computer programs, computerized record linkage can now be conducted on microcomputers with widely available statistical packages, although it still requires a good deal of expert judgment to interpret the odds. There are obvious concerns for protection of privacy, since the files used were usually generated for a different purpose, but provision can be made to prevent abuses, e.g., by having the entire matching process carried out within the statistical agency, and giving the investigator only summary data. I am not aware of any cases in which use of computerized record linkage for health research has resulted in the invasion of privacy (Newcombe, 1995).

3.3 Population (Denominator) Data

Population data play a more important role in policy epidemiology than in etiological research because policy happens in real-world populations, not in specially selected research populations. Demographic changes are enormously important in this respect, and there is no reason not to plan for them, since we know what the age–sex composition of the population will be for the next several decades. A recent popular book claims that demography explains "two-thirds of everything," from shoe sales to land values (Foot, 1996). An epidemiologic phenomenon can be important either because it is very marked or because it affects a segment of the population that is large or growing (cf. population attributable fraction). Sociodemographic data are needed for describing the population, estimating trends, and calculating rates, and are often determinants of health in their own right (e.g., income, education, occupation).

The Census

The most important source of population data is the census. Most countries conduct regular censuses at 10-year intervals; a less complete 5-year census may also be conducted. By definition a census is a count of the entire population (in contrast to a sample survey), although censuses may use sampling for detailed questions. Although census geography varies by country, two units are common to many censuses. The *enumeration district* (*enumeration area, block group*) is the group of households visited by a single census enumerator, numbering about 200; usually no results are released for these small areas. The *census tract* is a relatively homogeneous area with a population of 4000–5000, sometimes defined only in urban areas, and is the smallest unit for which results are normally available. Census tracts aggregate to municipalities, counties, etc., as well as electoral constituencies. Missing data may be replaced by imputation, i.e., the average value of a missing variable in similar individuals or households may be inserted. Results may be rounded before publication, and various forms of data suppression used to protect privacy. For example, in the 1991 Census of Canada (Statistics Canada, 1992:188) all numbers were randomly rounded (up or down) to a multiple of 5, with the result that columns of figures do not add to their reported totals. Furthermore, all data were suppressed for areas with a population less than 40, as were variables containing income information for areas with a population less than 250. Additional rules applied for suppression of individual cells.

Census data are usually made available in the form of tables of aggregate data, with relatively few categories and few cross-tabulations. It may be possible to purchase special tables, customized to the users' needs, subject to privacy rules. Microdata files are available in the form of random samples of the national census data file, which allow users to carry out their own analyses. Although the census theoretically covers the entire population (by law), there is in fact substantial undercounting of some population groups, e.g., young black males in the United States and aboriginals in Canada. These errors may be as high as 20% for some subgroups. Published data may be "corrected" for this undercount, although the correction can only be imperfect.

Postcensal and intercensal estimates

The appearance of census data at only 5 or 10-year intervals causes several problems. Annual population data are often needed for planning, marketing, and evaluating policies and programs. Annual mortality and morbidity rates are also desirable to detect short-term trends and impress media and policymakers with the recency of data. Numerator data appear every year, but equivalent denominator data are lacking. The most recent census data are sometimes used for the ensuing 5 to 10-year period, but this can produce distorted results: when a population is growing, the numerator events increase, but if the denominator data do not grow, the calculated rates will make it appear that the disease being investigated is becoming more common, even if it is quite stable (see example in Box 3–1).

To fill the need for very recent and for annual data, population estimates are produced by various levels of government for past and current single years. *Postcensal total population estimates* are produced for each year following the most recent census, based on the "component method":

$$\text{Population}_{t+1} = \text{Population}_t + \text{Births}_t - \text{Deaths}_t + \text{Net Migration}_t$$

Preliminary, updated, and final versions may be issued, balancing users' needs for both timely and accurate estimates. Since single-year estimates

---

Box 3-1. The importance of postcensal estimates

A provincial Ministry of Health distributed the following data to local health planners, using the most recent census population for denominators for each of the succeeding years. The hospital separation data for one jurisdiction showed a steadily climbing hospitalization rate, despite efforts to stabilize it.

Year	Separations	Population (1986 census)	Rate/1000	Population (postcensal estimate)	Rate/1000
1986	68,877	619,049	111.3	619,049	111.3
1987	70,412	619,049	113.7	633,349	111.2
1988	71,230	619,049	115.1	647,979	109.9
1989	72,197	619,049	116.6	662,948	108.9
Ratio (1989/1986)			1.05		0.98

When (admittedly crude) intercensal population estimates were later substituted for the 1986 Census population, an apparent 5% increase in the hospital separation rate over a 3-year period proved to be actually a slight decrease, which is a very different message for health planners concerned about hospital utilization rates. Use of postcensal estimates would have reduced or eliminated the problem in the first place.

---

are often used as the basis for grants from senior levels of government and for marketing purposes (e.g., attracting businesses to a community), municipalities and regions producing their own estimates may be tempted to make high estimates. Migration at regional levels can be very rapid, following trends in the economy, and is not well recorded. Therefore, estimates for regions and especially for smaller areas tend to be much less accurate than those for the country as a whole. More sophisticated regression modeling techniques are sometimes used to estimate the populations of small areas for single years, incorporating "symptomatic indicators," such as data from school boards and drivers' licenses (Statistics Canada, 1990).

More accurate *intercensal estimates* are produced for each year, after the next census results are available. The postcensal estimates are retrospectively adjusted, based on the *error of closure*, which is the difference between the most recent census count (the benchmark) and the postcensal estimate for the census year. Cruder estimates can be derived simply by interpolating between two censuses; the interpolations should usually use a log scale, since uniform relative changes are more likely than uniform absolute changes. Aickin et al. (1991) report more accurate results from regressing the logarithms of census counts on polynomials in time, e.g.,

$$\ln(\text{population}) = \beta_0 + \beta_1 t + \beta_2 t^2 + \beta_3 t^3$$

Other Sources of Population Data

Since a census is conducted only every 5–10 years, and there is significant lag time to publication, census data are out of date most of the time. Other sources of data may help to fill this gap. Several different government agencies may possess relatively complete administrative data. In countries with universal health insurance programs, the list of beneficiaries for these plans may be fairly complete, since individuals have a strong incentive to ensure that they are registered. Voters' lists may be useful, although they list only adults eligible to vote and provide little information about them. Municipal tax rolls list the population, although they may exclude children and tenants. And of course, income tax is inevitable. Statistics Canada has developed the T1 Family File database (T1FF) (Lucaciu, 1993) from personal income tax forms as a source of timely annual population data. Tax returns are linked to one another to identify spouses and grown children, and dependents are identified from parents' returns; year of birth of children is either looked up in the Family Allowance File or imputed from the mother's age, but sex is not known for imputed children's records. The resulting T1FF is published annually, about 18 months after the date to which it refers. Coverage is claimed to be excellent (97% overall), and is improving as more people file tax returns to collect social benefits, even if they are not required to pay any tax. Variables are obviously limited to those included on the tax return: family type and size, age, sex, address, amount and sources of income, employment status and language in which the form is completed. An evaluation found the database to be reasonably accurate, especially in urban areas, but lamented its cost and the delays in its release (Spasoff and Gilkes, 1994).

Population Registers

Some countries, e.g., Scandinavian countries and The Netherlands, maintain registers of the population in each municipality. In The Netherlands, this reflects the unwillingness of the population to participate in a census, which has therefore not been conducted for many years. Residents have a legal responsibility to be on the register, which therefore contains up-to-date information but a limited numbers of variables. Access to the register is permitted to legitimate investigators and agencies. In principle, such a register provides the ideal denominator for calculation of rates and an excellent sampling frame for surveys or case–control studies.

Population Projections

The characteristics of tomorrow's population are as important to health policy makers and planners as are those of today's population. A *population projection* is a mathematical calculation of what the future population might be, given alternative, plausible assumptions about future fertility, mortality and migration (Ministry of Treasury and Economics, 1989). In contrast to postcensal estimates, which concern the present and the very recent past, population projections refer to the future, but the same basic formula applies. In general, only age and sex breakdowns are provided. Statistics Canada produces projections for the next 30 years that are based on various assumptions regarding fertility (high, medium, low), mortality, internal migration, and international migration (high, low) (Statistics Canada, 1990). Migration is the most difficult to quantify. Changes in fertility are sufficiently unpredictable that projections beyond 5 years or so must be treated with great caution. As with single-year estimates, it is often in the interests of local jurisdictions to make self-enhancing projections.

3.4 Health (Numerator) Data

These data are counts of health events or states, such as death, disease, hospitalization, or visit to the doctor.

Disease Classifications

If interest extends beyond the fact of an event to the nature of the event, some classification is essential. Several are in common use, four of which are noted here.

The *International Statistical Classification of Diseases and Related Health Problems* (ICD; World Health Organization, 1992) is used internationally and is now in its 10th revision (although North America was still using the 9th revision in 1998). The ICD-10 provides a 4-digit code for each disease or condition and is arranged in 21 chapters. Originally designed for classifying causes of death, it still works best for categorizing deaths and hospitalizations, where the diagnosis is usually fairly clear; when used for coding primary care utilization, a high proportion of all visits end up being coded very uncomfortably in residual categories. A peculiarity of the ICD is the number of different dimensions represented by its chapters, which relate variously to cause (infectious disease), pathology (neoplasms), body system (respiratory, etc.), and manifestations (symptoms). Two separate sets of codes are provided for injuries: external cause and nature of injury. Proposals have been made for a more general two-dimensional classification, but to date this possibility exists only to a very limited extent for other conditions. Such a change would allow the coding of conditions like "tobacco disease," the estimation of which currently requires considerable manipulation of the data, using population attributable fractions. More fundamental criticisms of the ICD are that it is excessively influenced by the medical culture with its emphasis on disease, and that it cannot deal with health or its social and environmental determinants (Stallones, 1980).

The *International Classification for Primary Care* (ICPC; Lamberts and Wood, 1987) recognizes that the problems presenting in primary care are relatively undifferentiated, and also provides much more scope for coding psychological and social problems. It is divided into 17 chapters on one axis, organ-systems, and seven components on the other axis: symptoms and complaints, five aspects of process of care, and diagnosis. It can be used in several modes: reason for encounter, diagnosis, or process. All of its codes can be translated into the ICD through a computer program.

The *International Classification of Impairment, Disability and Handicap* (ICIDH; World Health Organization, 1980) acknowledges that the nature of a limitation is often more important than its cause. Its major contribution has been to clarify the distinction between the following:

- Impairment: "any loss or abnormality of psychological, physiological, or anatomical structure or function," e.g., cataracts, amputations
- Disability: "any restriction or lack (resulting from an impairment) of ability to perform an activity in the manner or within the range considered normal for a human being," e.g., blindness, inability to walk
- Handicap: "disadvantage for a given individual, resulting from an impairment or disability that limits or prevents the fulfillment of a role that is normal (depending on age, sex, and social and cultural factors) for that individual," e.g., student, construction worker.

The classification acknowledges that disability is determined by an individual's psychological makeup and the rehabilitation services received as well as by impairment, and that handicap depends as much the physical and social environment as the individual. Disability and handicap provide a highly integrated or "summary" assessment of an individual's health, which for policy purposes is often more useful than a specific diagnosis.

The *Diagnostic and Statistical Manual for Mental Disorders* (DSM; American Psychiatric Association, 1994), currently in its 4th version (DSM-IV), was developed in response to the difficulty in establishing psychiatric diagnoses and the poor reliability among different physicians in doing so. It is exemplary in that it provides detailed diagnostic criteria and is translatable into the ICD.

Postal Code Conversion

Postal code conversion is an essential tool for public health and policy research, at least in some countries. Most health numerator data have addresses coded according to postal geography. These tend to be hierarchical, with the first few characters indicating geographic regions and the later characters specifying neighborhood, street, or even building. The most commonly used denominator data come from the census and are organized according to census geography (census tracts, municipalities, electoral districts), raising the need to convert one set of geographic codes to the other. Ultimately, it might be best to use postal code geography for all purposes. But census tracts have been defined to be relatively homogeneous, making them useful for public health planning, and they aggregate to the geopolitical boundaries that are often relevant to health policy. Therefore, policy researchers usually prefer to use census geography and try to convert numerator data to it. The issue may eventually be resolved by introduction of *geographic information systems* (GIS; Scholten and de Lepper, 1991), which allow very detailed geographic coding of any variable; this system is currently being introduced in many jurisdictions.

A postal code conversion file is needed to convert postal codes to census geography. Street index programs are also available for converting street addresses directly to census geography, but many recorded addresses are inexact because of spelling errors, confusion between streets and avenues, etc., so postal code conversions are more practical. The conversions work well at high levels of aggregation (provinces and large regions), but less well for lower levels. Similarly (in Canada), postal code conversion works very well in urban areas, where postal codes are geographically small, but much less well in rural areas, where a single postal code may overlap several census tracts and even several municipalities, and the user must find some way to assign each postal code to a single census unit.

Privacy Protection

Statistical agencies have rules governing release of data. For example, Statistics Canada specifies that an estimate can be used without qualification if its coefficient of variation (CV) < 16.5% and published with caution if $16.5\% \leq CV \leq 33.3\%$, but should not be released if CV > 33.3% (Stephens and Fowler Graham, 1993). Especially for dichotomous variables, the sample sizes (or equivalently, the number of events) required to achieve these values can be quite discouraging, as shown in Table 3-2 for several values of p. It follows that data suppression occurs frequently when the sample is small, when looking at subgroups, or when the occurrence is rare in the population. This is frustrating for the user, as these are often the data of particular interest, but it is important to resist the temptation to use such unstable estimates.

Uses, Availability, and Quality of Data

Vital statistics

Vital statistics are at the core of health data and have the advantage of being available for the entire population. They can help to define high-

Table 3-2. Required Sample Size for Data Release

p	CV = 16.5%		CV = 33%	
	No. of Events	Sample Size	No. of Events	Sample Size
0.001	37	36,694	9	9,174
0.01	36	3,636	9	909
0.1	33	331	8	83
0.5	18	37	5	9

Source: Calculated from Statistics Canada guidelines (Stephens and Fowler Graham, 1993:15).

risk areas and can support ecological research (e.g., on the effects of socioeconomic factors on birth and death rates).

Natality data can be used to measure fertility and birth rates and the frequency of various reproductive outcomes such as low birth weight, stillbirths, and preterm birth. Virtually all live births and stillbirths are registered in developed countries. No complete data are available for spontaneous abortions, although data for legally induced abortions are available. Usually the attending health professional records data for each birth on a special form, which is sent to the responsible government agency. The form includes data on both the mother (identification, age, postal code, marital status, occupation, number of previous live births and stillbirths) and the infant(s) (place of birth, year/month/day of birth, sex, weight, gestation period, live or stillbirth, singleton or multiple birth, congenital anomalies). Not all of these data are necessarily released. There is a tendency to round the birth weight up to 2500 g, the usual cut-off for low birth weight. Non-standard coding and data entry procedures can make comparisons across regions untrustworthy.

Mortality data quantify the ultimate health problems: those which cause death. These are thus the "hardest" health data, as there is little doubt about the fact of death, and as virtually all deaths are recorded in developed countries. Indeed, the main reason that they are the most widely used "health" data is their universal availability. But mortality is an insensitive indicator of health. Most of the feasible improvements have already been made in many countries, which may be near the irreducible minimum mortality. Many important causes of morbidity, such as mental and musculoskeletal diseases, rarely cause death. But the classic epidemiologic approach is to deplore the use the use of mortality statistics because of their diagnostic inaccuracy and insensitivity to the health of the living, and then proceed to use them on the grounds that at least they are available. They are often used as proxies for morbidity, on the assumption that mortality has similar causes and distributions to morbidity. Access to the data can be a major problem, since statistical agencies may not release data below a certain level (in Canada the lowest kind is municipalities—regardless of their population!), effectively preventing any analysis of small-area variations.

The key step in generating mortality data is the earliest and least controlled one: completion of the death certificate by a physician. Cause of death is often incompletely or inaccurately recorded by physicians, and coding is not uniform across various jurisdictions (Balkau et al., 1993). Since only the underlying cause of death is coded in many jurisdictions, associated diseases that contribute to death but that tend not to cause death directly (e.g., diabetes) tend to be underrecorded. Addresses may be incorrect, as persons from outlying areas may list their address as the largest nearby town instead of their own township or village. As the example in Box 3-2 shows, this can inflate the apparent death rates for towns and deflate those for the surrounding rural areas.

Morbidity

The term "morbidity" is used here rather generally to refer to the incidence and prevalence of diseases, presence of impairment, disability, or

---

Box 3-2. The (apparent) hazards of living in small places

The third volume of the *Mortality Atlas of Canada* (Health and Welfare Canada and Statistics Canada, 1984) presents standardized mortality ratios (SMRs) for all municipalities with a population greater than 5,000. In the initial results, the highest SMR in the country (at 1.8) was in Maniwaki, a small community 100 km north of the national capital. Local politicians were concerned about the impact on the town's ability to attract industry, while residents were convinced that it was the poor quality of the hospital and medical care, and public health officials pointed to the high unemployment and the heavy use of tobacco and alcohol. But epidemiologists found it strange that the SMRs were elevated for virtually every cause and suspected some sort of bias. A quick check revealed that the SMRs for the surrounding rural townships were even lower than those for Maniwaki were high: around 0.2. Examination of death certificates confirmed that residents of the rural townships tended to list their addresses as Maniwaki when admitted to hospital, and that this very approximate address found its way to their death certificates, while the denominator data (from the census) listed the addresses correctly. When the town and the surrounding townships were lumped together, the SMR was around 1.4, consistent with the depressed economy of the area. This value was confirmed after manual correction of the addresses on the individual birth certificates (Mao et al., 1984). The lumping procedure was subsequently applied to all small towns before the data were released.

handicap, and self-reported health. Morbidity data are much more relevant to health policy and planning than are mortality data, but they are also much less available. While the fact of death is clear, morbidity is multidimensional, partly subjective, and accordingly, hard to measure.

Diseases. Disease data are useful for assessing health status, identifying high-risk groups, and evaluating control programs. In the interests of disease control, certain communicable diseases are designated as *notifiable* (reportable) (Teutsch and Churchill, 1994); the list of notifiable diseases varies by jurisdiction. Public health acts require physicians and laboratories to report these diseases to the public health authorities. Although reporting is mandatory, it is incomplete to a varying extent; designating more diseases as notifiable could conceivably result in less complete reporting of each. However, the data are generally adequate to permit monitoring of trends. Cancer is the only noncommunicable disease for which population incidence data are widely available in most countries, as a product of cancer registries (Band et al., 1993), although these often do not cover a whole country. Most registries depend upon reporting by hospitals, physicians, and laboratories, but the Ontario Cancer Registry is generated entirely by record linkage of mortality, hospital, laboratory, and cancer clinic files (Clarke et al., 1987). Variables commonly include patient age, sex and address, site and stage of cancer, and survival status (confirmed through linkage with the mortality file, a process known as "death clearance"). Incidence and mortality data are available by age, sex, residence, site of cancer, and stage. The unit of analysis is usually the new primary cancer, not the individual. Most cancers are rare, and the small numbers mean that data may not be released in the detail that local users may desire. A delicate aggregation process is then required, balancing aggregation by site, geographic area, age and/or calendar year against the resulting loss of detail (dilution of patterns, obscuring of trends). Public health-care systems that are highly organized may generate data for a wider range of diseases, e.g., Lithuania has a country-wide diabetes registry that is generated by its diabetes clinics.

Impairment, disability and handicap. Impairment is fairly similar to disease, and the same data issues apply. Disability and handicap data omit diagnostic information, which is often imprecise or unhelpful, in favor of functional and social status, which is often more relevant to quality of life. This information is usually available only from health surveys, although investigators in Manitoba have attempted to estimate it from diagnoses drawn from utilization data (Cohen and MacWilliam, 1995). In some cases, employment disability data may be useful, although these are bound to be affected by the eligibility criteria for sick pay.

Health-related quality of life (see Section 3.1) provides a more sensitive measure of health because its components are relatively frequent, and it taps into the concept of positive health. But many of the required data are available only from sample surveys.

Self-reported health refers to symptoms, untreated morbidity, self-rated health status, and health knowledge, beliefs, attitudes, and behaviors. This valuable information is available only from surveys, and thus is limited by small sample sizes, irregular or infrequent conduct of surveys, and lack of comparability of methods.

Determinants of health/risk factors

Data are needed for both population-level and individual-level factors to assess health risks and needs, target and evaluate risk factor intervention programs, and predict future health. They are of widely differing availability. *Demographic* risk factors appear as part of the population data discussed above and provide the substrate in which health phenomena occur. Other risk factors can be classified by their proximity to the health events, ranging from proximal to distal.

Physiological risk factors, such as blood pressure, cholesterol level, and immune status, are closest to the health events. They are generally available only from household surveys that incorporate physical measures, e.g., the National Health and Nutrition Examination Survey (NHANES) in the United States, and thus are comparatively sparse. Measurement of *genetic* risk factors requires more specialized laboratory facilities; they will become more important in the near future, with the findings from the Human Genome Project.

Behavioral risk factors, such as smoking and alcohol consumption, are generally available at the individual level from health surveys, e.g., the National Health Interview Survey and the Behavioral Risk Factor Surveillance System in the United States. They are obviously subject to inaccurate reporting, although the technology for asking the appropriate questions is highly developed, and the results are occasionally validated by objective (e.g., biochemical) measures. Diet is notoriously difficult to quantify through interview. Frequency questionnaires and 24-hour or 1-week recall questionnaires compete with diaries as the most appropriate measurement method (Willett 1998). Collection of data on physical activity presents similar problems. Another approach (for tobacco, alcohol, and specific foods) uses consumption data, but these apply only to the population in general, without breakdowns for specific groups, and do not reflect cross-border consumption or smuggling.

Most remote from health events and influencing the all other risk factors are *environmental* risk factors. Data for the physical environment are generally collected on an ecological basis (except in the rare cases where personal monitors are available, as for radiation exposure and occasionally for air pollution) and are notoriously difficult to relate to health status data because individuals move through many microenvironments each day. Further developments in geographic information systems (GIS) may help to resolve these problems. Data for the social environment, e.g., social support, present similar conceptual problems and are often even harder to measure.

Health services
Data are needed for the supply and utilization of institutions (hospitals, nursing homes, clinics, laboratories) and health professionals (physicians, dentists, nurses, physiotherapists). Relative to health status and risk factors, a wealth of information is available, although it tends not to be population based or person oriented.

Supply. Health-policy makers need to know the numbers and nature of health resources, their distribution, and their activity status (e.g., the nature of services provided and whether professionals are working full-time). Data on the supply of hospital beds are readily available, but with the move toward ambulatory care, the number of beds has become less meaningful as an indicator of a hospital's capacity. It is important to distinguish between total and staffed (operating) beds; not all beds are available for use. More fundamentally, the definition of hospital is changing, and mergers make the counting of individual institutions more difficult. Furthermore, it is often difficult to relate supply to population needs, as hospital catchment populations are rarely defined.

Long-term care is harder to quantify because of the range in levels of care, the different classifications used by different jurisdictions, and the ill-defined boundary between long-term care and housing. Data on community health services are even more difficult to quantify because of their diversity and the lack of any widely accepted unit of measurement or capacity, as well as the ill-defined boundary between community health and social services. The numbers of regulated health professionals, including doctors, dentists, and registered nurses, are available from licensing authorities, but their practice location or status, i.e., full-or part-time, specialist or generalist, may not be. The latter information is remarkably hard to obtain because status frequently changes and many professionals work outside institutional settings. Unregulated health professionals are even harder to define and count.

Utilization. The availability of utilization data depends greatly upon the organization of the health-care system, particularly upon payment arrangements. Such data are important measures of the functioning of the health-care system, for they help assess access, detect abuses, and plan locations of services. They are often used as surrogates of morbidity for conditions that are almost always treated. The Nova Scotia–Saskatchewan Heart Study linked hospital and mortality data to estimate the incidence of acute myocardial infarction in these provinces (Nova Scotia–Saskatchewan Cardiovascular Disease Epidemiology Group, 1989);

obviously these data address only hospitalized morbidity, not that treated on an ambulatory basis or not treated at all. The potential exists for similar achievements in other diseases. But the use of utilization data to measure morbidity calls for great caution because utilization is determined by many factors other than need (e.g., supply, health insurance provisions, and provider and consumer habits). It is a well-established principle of health care research that available hospital beds will be filled—the "availability effect" first described by Roemer (1961)—so a population that is well supplied with hospital beds will look sicker by measures based on utilization than one that is less well supplied (certain North American cities have since shown that there are limits beyond which utilization cannot be pushed). The same pattern has been found for physicians. Use of utilization data to define needs tends to perpetuate existing patterns of care. Hospitals send abstracts of separations (effectively the same as admissions) to a central abstracting service, which prepares profiles of the care provided in individual hospitals and summaries of data across hospitals. The system may cover acute hospitals, chronic hospitals, nursing homes and homes for the aged, with or without day surgery, emergency and out-patient visits. Patient variables include age, birth date, sex, address, and health insurance number (which may be scrambled to avoid revealing the identity of a subject, but consistently so, rendering multiple admissions of the same patient identifiable as such, if the insurance numbers are correctly recorded on all admissions). Institutional variables may identify the admitting institution as well as those from which the patient was transferred and to which the patient was discharged, if any. Illness variables are of relatively high quality and may include several diagnostic codes (which are normally ICD; the U.S. uses an adaptation of these), most responsible diagnosis for the hospital stay, admission diagnosis, complications, some measure of intensity of care, and procedures. Tables are available for both separations and days of care; microdata may also be available. These files are very large, placing heavy demands on expertise, hardware, and software. More important, records generally refer to hospitalizations, not to individuals, and it may be difficult to obtain unduplicated counts of persons and therefore to determine disease incidence. Access to these data is severely limited by provisions for the protection of privacy: to preserve hospital confidentiality, data may be released only for aggregations of several hospitals. In the United States, the Health Care Cost and Utilization Project of the Agency for Health Care Policy and Research makes both nationwide and state data available from a 20% sample of hospitals.

Utilization of physicians' services is more problematic. Since patients have short memories and physicians have inconsistent records, insurance records are usually the best source of information. The availability of utilization data therefore depends on the nature and scope of health insurance: a single insurer (as in the Canadian provinces) can generate uniform data for a whole population more readily than a host of insurers (as in the U.S.), who will have different procedures and may be unwilling to disclose their data for business reasons. While some jurisdictions (notably the Canadian province of Manitoba, as described in Section 3.5) have set up their insurance plans to generate epidemiologically useful data, others fall abysmally short of this level. At best, they record information about reason for medical visit, diagnosis, and services provided, although there are major concerns, expressed especially by physicians, about the quality of the diagnostic data. At worst, insurance records may indicate only total expenditures for physicians' services, perhaps broken down by provider and by age and sex of the patients. The Ontario health insurance plan failed to record its beneficiaries individually or provide them with unique identifying numbers, the result being that the denominator could never be clearly defined (and eventually came to include over 20 million individuals in a population of 10 million). In the United States, the Medical Expenditures Panel Survey provides an alternative source of information based on longitudinal samples of households, medical providers, insurance plans, and nursing homes. Population-based information on utilization of prescription drugs is available for the province of Saskatchewan through its universal drug plan. Information on utilization of other personal health services is normally available only from population health surveys. Public health services often have their own information systems that are unlinked to those for personal health services. Utilization data for community health services are the least adequate of all, as they are often provided by poorly funded organizations whose administrators believe that they have better things to do than collect data.

Costs of care. Global data for total health care expenditures are compiled by governments from a variety of sources and published as absolute amounts and percentage of the gross domestic product (GDP). Data on the costs of care for individual patients are harder to come by and are complicated by issues similar to those concerning utilization. One cannot assume that the average per-diem cost of hospital care reflects the true costs of caring for an individual patient: some patients require far more expensive care than others, and the cost of care for an individual patient is usually much higher in the early than in the later days of a hospitalization (so that shortening length of stay eliminates cheap days). Hospital accounting systems in the United States quantify the costs of care for individual patients as part of billing procedures, and diagnosis-related groups (DRGs) provide a convenient unit of observation. Canadian hospitals have traditionally been paid by global budgets and have generated no data on the costs of caring for individual patients, but the development of case-mix groups (equivalent to DRGs) and associated relative intensity weights allows more accurate estimation of the costs of a patient's stay.

For physicians' services, the situation is again determined by the payment provisions. Under universal medical care insurance, such data are based on payments to individual physicians, and where payment is fee-for-service it is often possible to relate the payments to patients and problems. In the absence of universal insurance, data may be available from surveys of patients or providers, but the former are likely to be inaccurate and the latter fail to relate the expenditures to the characteristics of consumers or their health problems.

Quality of care. The efficacy (potential effectiveness) of health care interventions is the subject of much of the health care and clinical epidemiology literature, but their actual effectiveness (in the field) remains largely undocumented by routinely collected data. Statistics on hospital readmissions and on complications of care are relevant but are rather limited in their ability to measure quality of care (Lohr, 1988). In the United States, the Health Plan Employer Data and Information Set (HEDIS) database provides performance indicators for health maintenance organizations.

3.5 A Population Health Information System

Purposes

The first step in converting health information into health intelligence is its assembly into a population health information system. Such a system can then be used to

- develop profiles of a population's health;
- identify problems or groups in need of interventions;
- identify threats to the public health;
- evaluate health policy in terms of the effects on the public's health of the investments made.

It should support better decisions regarding the planning, implementation, and evaluation of health programs and thereby make these programs more responsive to needs and more effective. Ultimately, it should improve the population's health. In addition, health information is relatively cheap, compared to the total economic burden of ill health or the amount spent on health services. As already noted, the field of information science has not been well tapped for the purpose of developing population-based systems. Friede et al. (1995) have called for the development of a discipline of public health informatics, which they define as "the application of information science and technology to public health practice and research." The concept encompasses data systems, information systems, and communications. There is a long way to go to achieve their vision.

Sponsorship

Development of a community health information system involves a partnership between government and local agencies such as public health units and health planning councils, as well as health professionals and institutions. Local agencies are increasingly the users of the data, but they usually lack the expertise and resources to do the work themselves. Governments must therefore provide both administrative and financial support. Government is the source of many of the data and is in a position to coordinate health information activities. Without such coordination, different areas are likely to develop incompatible information systems and generate noncomparable data. Maintaining the actual health database seems inherently a public function to be undertaken by government or perhaps (in these days of smaller government) on behalf of government. Any statistical agency that is required to be financially self-supporting will inevitably end up serving only industry and large institutions (mainly drug companies and hospitals), and its products are unlikely to benefit the whole population. Marketing and education are important supporting functions if local agencies are to use such a database. Agencies must clearly demonstrate the benefits of having health information collected and accessible if the public and politicians are to be informed and supportive. Health intelligence units have been developed in Ontario to facilitate use of data at the local level (Neufeld and Spasoff, 1992); these units are sponsored by health planning councils, public health agencies and academic health sciences centers, and funded by the provincial government.

Attributes

Wolfson (1992) describes a "health information template" or conceptual framework that is very comprehensive and intuitive but which appears to exist only in conceptual form (see Fig. 3-3). To the extent that such a system were to cover the entire population, it would allow individual-based analyses, linking individual records from different sources as well as summary breakdowns. To the extent that the system were to use data based on samples (e.g., health survey data), it would allow descriptive studies as well as specialized studies of the sample members for whom data were available, e.g., follow-up of respondents to a health survey, which would usually be satisfactory.

It is assumed, however, that linked microdata will not be available in the near future in most jurisdictions and that the available aggregate data will be organized by geographic area. The geographic areas should conform to administrative boundaries, most likely census tracts, which aggregate to municipalities and counties. Data should be broken down at least by age and sex. Ideally, all the data types noted in Section 3.4 should be represented.

An outstanding example of a population health information system is found in Box 3-3.

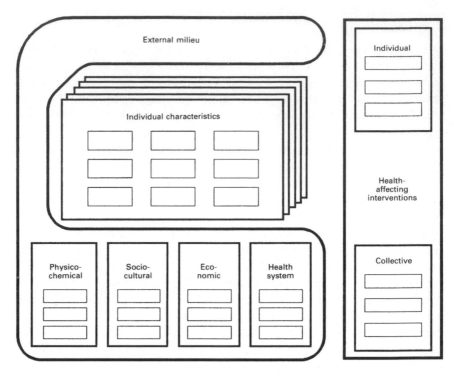

Figure 3-3. Health information template. [From Wolfson, 1992:111.]

Box 3-3. Manitoba's POPULIS

Manitoba's Population Health Information System, POPULIS (Roos and Shapiro, 1995), is a highly developed system based on administrative data. Using the conceptual model of health that was developed in the population health movement (Fig. 3-2; Evans and Stoddart, 1994), the system incorporates data on vital statistics, hospital and nursing home utilization, physicians' services and prescribed drugs from a population of one million. These data can then be related to census data on an ecological basis. The use of health insurance data is greatly facilitated by the presence of universal government health insurance, and the use of a single health insurance number for all health services has allowed linkage of databases arising from different sources. Software has been developed for record linkage and analysis. The system has been used to study health needs, inequalities in health, resource allocation, small-area variations in health care, adverse effects of health care, and consequences of closing hospital beds.

Summary

Health is multidimensional and dynamic and tends to defy operational definition. Although the existence of positive health is generally acknowledged, most operational definitions are built on freedom from disease. Health data need to be analyzed to produce health information and then interpreted to form health intelligence, upon which rational decisions can be based. Computerized record linkage enables the use of administrative data for studying the health and health care of entire populations, but raises concerns regarding protection of privacy. Routinely collected data such as vital statistics are at least as relevant as data specially collected by research projects. Aggregated data (based on groups) do not permit reconstruction of the characteristics of any individual; they also require somewhat different techniques from those used for microdata (data referring to individuals). Although peripheral to etiological research, population data are central to policy epidemiology. Denominator data are usually obtained from the census, necessitating a knowledge of census methods and geography. Postcensal and intercensal estimates are needed to assess health trends and can range from simple interpolation to complex techniques using other sources of information. Population projections are needed for predicting future developments; this is one of many areas to which demography makes a vital contribution to health policy. Other sources of information, such as taxation data or population registers, may sometimes supplement or even replace the census. Numerator data are more varied. Disease classifications are necessary to make health data meaningful; four are relevant here: ICD, ICPC, ICIDH, and DSM. Although most denominator data are organized according to administrative geography, many numerator data are coded according to postal address, making postal code conversion an essential skill. Availability and quality of health data vary widely by type and jurisdiction. A population health information system should contain data on population, mortality, morbidity, risk factors, and health services. Ideally, these would be available for individuals (microdata); they must at least be linkable to geographic areas.

Key References

Friede A, Blum HL, McDonald M. Public Health Informatics: How information-age technology can strengthen public health. *Annu Rev Public Health* 1995;16:239–52.

Roos NP, Shapiro E (eds.) Health and health care: experience with a population-based health information system. *Med Care* 1995;33(12) (Suppl): DS1–DS146.

Wolfson MC. A template for health information. *World Health Stat Q* 1992; 45:109–113.

II

THE POLICY CYCLE

Epidemiology can contribute to each step of the policy cycle:

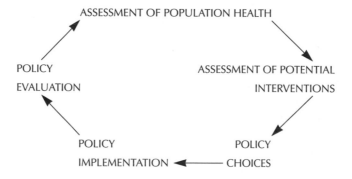

Each of the remaining chapters of this book is devoted to one of these steps.

4

Assessment of Population Health

With the community health database in place, it is time to consider its uses. Development of population health profiles is a major one. How healthy is the population? Is its health getting better or worse? Are some areas or subgroups much healthier than others? How can we quantify these differences? What is the impact of ill health on society? How can we measure this? What are the population's health needs? What risks does it face? What explains the differences in health? This chapter begins the process of converting health information into health intelligence.

4.1 Developing a Population Health Profile

Scope and Purpose

A population health profile is a summary of the health of a defined population. It might be used to support development or review of health policy, a health goals process, a needs assessment for health programs, or resource allocation. Production of periodic health reports is mandatory in many jurisdictions to monitor progress in improving or maintaining health.

Organizational Arrangements

Community members should be involved in developing health profiles. The process contributes to empowerment of the population, ensures that the profile covers the topics of interest to the community, and enables use of the special knowledge of the community that residents bring. It also educates community members about health issues (thereby building a constituency for subsequent action) and epidemiologists about public priorities.

Unit of analysis

Sometimes the interest is in a jurisdiction as a whole, but often there is interest in making comparisons among subareas. How large should these subareas be, in terms of population? Ideally, they should be small enough to be relatively internally homogeneous but large enough to provide stable rates and avoid cell suppression when acquiring data. The actual numbers will depend on the data breakdowns desired. Both the data sources and the eventual uses dictate that administrative jurisdictions be used as much as possible. Municipalities vary too much in size to be useful as the sole unit of analysis; cities are very heterogeneous and always need to be sub-subdivided, while rural municipalities are too small. Census tracts are too small for most purposes (the average population is about 5000): numerator events are too rare to yield stable rates, and agencies will not release data for such small groups. Electoral wards or other relevant subareas have been administratively defined in some cities, but in other cases it may be necessary to create intermediate areas or "neighborhoods": aggregations of contiguous census tracts, all within the same municipality, with fairly similar characteristics and populations around 20,000. For studying rare conditions like cancer, it may be necessary to create larger aggregations, with a population of at least 50,000. Reasonable criteria for grouping census tracts are age, household composition, income, education, and ethnic group; expert advice should be obtained from organizations such as planning departments, public health units, and regional health councils. The needs of the participating agencies may be quite varied, requiring different aggregations for different purposes. Naturally, the larger the groupings, the more internally heterogeneous they become, concealing potentially important differences, and the more they become similar to one another. The United Kingdom Office of National Statistics has defined "area classification groups" as aggregations of areas with similar socioeconomic and demographic characteristics that are not geographically contiguous (National Institute of Epidemiology, 1997). They carry descriptive names like Coast & Country, Coalfields, and Growth Areas. Such aggregations are very useful for studying policy issues, e.g., inequalities in health (because the problems of using small numbers are avoided), but less so for planning and programming local health services.

Data Coverage

Relevant data may cover the entire population (the census), the entire affected population (vital statistics, cancer registries, hospital morbidity data), or only a sample of the population (health surveys). This distinction influences the feasibility of using various data in a health profile. When the population of interest is relatively small, e.g., census tracts, the census is the only data source with adequate sample size to support development of the profile. The census can provide sociodemographic data relevant to the determinants of health, including age, sex, ethnic group, language, household composition, education, and income. But beyond this level of description, it may only be possible to make assumptions about health status (or to attempt small-area estimation, as described below). Although mortality, hospital morbidity, and cancer incidence data exist for the whole affected population, they are not usable for very small areas because the affected segment is too small. Data on untreated morbidity or risk factors are available only for fairly large populations because of the limited sample size in health surveys. Various forms of aggregation are then necessary to achieve access to the data, e.g., broader age-groups or diagnostic categories, or larger geographic areas.

Population Health Indicators

As noted in Chapter 1, the terms "public health" and "population health" are sometimes used to refer to the health of the public or the population. But is the health of a population different from the aggregated health of the individuals who comprise it (Rose, 1985)? Health promoters would argue that it is, but others find the separate specification of the population level useful only for determinants of health. Either way, the profile will need health indicators to summarize data and facilitate comparisons among jurisdictions and groups.

The term *health indicator* seems to convey two related ideas. First, an indicator is a variable used as a proxy for a variable that cannot be measured directly: "A health indicator is a variable, susceptible to direct measurement, that reflects the state of health of persons in a community" (Last, 1995:74). All the examples provided are summary measures, such as rates. Measurements may be either direct expressions of what they are intended to measure or indirect measures that are correlated with direct measures; utilization of health services is a direct measure of utilization, but is also used as an indirect measure of health status (Rosén, 1987: 54). It is debatable whether any direct measurements of health exist, with the possible exception of self-rated health. Other definitions of health indicators emphasize their summarizing function across individuals: "[S]tatistics selected from the larger pool because they have the power to summarize, to represent a larger body of statistics, or to serve as indirect or proxy measures for information that is lacking. . . . As a rule they represent or summarize one class of data only (e.g., mortality or morbidity but not the two together)" (Murnaghan, 1981:303). For clarity we shall distinguish between *individual health indicators* (the data in the cells of Table 4-1) and *population health indicators* (the statistics that appear in the bottom margin of the table). The latter rates, averages, proportions, and ratios are widely used in public health and policy analysis.

The choice of indicators of health status depends on the goals and objectives of a society. At present, most relate to mortality and morbidity, i.e., deviations from health. Indicators of equity and of positive health are particularly needed; it seems a little strained to use "absence of medical consumption" as an indicator of positive health (Ruwaard et al., 1994:36). It has been argued that the social sciences have the most to offer in this respect, and that increased use should be made of lay knowledge. In this view, epidemiology, public health, and health services research are too narrow, too committed to a biomedical model of health.

Table 4-1. Individual and Population Health

Individuals (ID#)	Dimensions of Health, with Examples			
	Mortality	Disability	Self-rated Health	Health Indices
	Age at death	Existence of disability	Self-rated health	
1				Individual health
2				indices
Population indicators	Life expectancy	Prevalence of disability	Average self-rating	Population health index

In Canada, the Community Health Information System project has developed a framework for community health information for public health services (Working Group on Community Health Information Systems, 1995), along with computer programs for manipulating community health data and calculating the indicators. Although developed for public health planning, its 60 indicators (summarized in Box 4-1) have wider relevance to health policy. Similar lists have been developed in other jurisdictions, e.g., the indicators used in the Healthy People initiative in the United States (Department of Health and Human Services, 1991) and the Public Health Common Data Set in the United Kingdom (National Institute of Epidemiology, 1997).

Population Health Indices

Health indices are often used to reduce the quantity and increase the interpretability of data. The Dictionary of Epidemiology defines a *health index* as "a numerical indication of the health of a given population derived from a specified composite formula. The components of the formula [are] . . . health indicators" (Last, 1995:74). Returning to Table 4-1, when individual health indicators are combined across dimensions, they yield *individual health indices* (right margin of the table), the wealth of which has been catalogued by McDowell and Newell (1996). Examples are the SF-36 (Ware and Sherbourne, 1992) and the Sickness Impact Profile (Bergner et al., 1981). Normally such indices cover only self-reported health, although some are quite wide-ranging. For example, the 36 questions of the SF-36 assess eight dimensions of health: physical functioning, role limitations due to physical health problems, bodily pain, social functioning, general mental health, role limitations due to emotional problems, vitality, and general perceptions. The EuroQol (EuroQol Group, 1990) and the McMaster Health Utility Index (Boyle et al., 1995) are designed to yield a single value for use in economic analyses; the Health Utility Index was incorporated into the Ontario Health Survey and the Canadian Na-

Box 4-1. Health status indicators: community health information systems (Working Group on Community Health Information Systems, 1995)

1. Determinants of health
1.1 Environment
1.1.1 Physical environment and ecology
> 3 indicators, e.g., proportion of population served by sewage treatment facilities

1.1.2 Social environment
> 3 demographic indicators, e.g., age-specific fertility rate
> 5 sociodemographic indicators, e.g., proportion of population living alone
> 6 socioeconomic indicators, e.g., unemployment rate

1.2 Human biology
> no indicators

1.3 Lifestyle, behaviors and risk factors
> 13 indicators, e.g., proportion of regular smokers

1.4 Organization of health care
> 5 indicators, e.g., average hospital stay by cause

2. Health status
2.1 Subjective health status
> 3 indicators, e.g., proportion who do not perceive themselves in good health

2.2 Objective health status
2.2.1 Non-hospital morbidity
> 3 indicators, e.g., incidence of notifiable diseases

2.2.2 Hospital morbidity
> 2 indicators, e.g., hospitalization rate by cause

2.2.3 Mortality
> 8 indicators, e.g., infant mortality rate

3. Consequences of health problems
3.1 Disability
> 3 indicators, e.g., proportion of children with handicaps

3.2 Use of services
> 4 indicators, e.g., medical consultation rate

3.3 Use of medication
> 2 indicators, e.g., annual number of prescription days for persons 65 or over

tional Population Health Surveys to permit longitudinal and geographic comparisons. Summarization across the population is a simple process of averaging to produce a *population health index*. In contrast to the major efforts on individual health indices, rather limited work has been done on combining population health indicators to form a population health index (bottom margin of Table 4-1; an example is quality-adjusted life expectancy in Section 2.2). Are the products of the row-first and column-first aggregations conceptually the same? Would they show similar patterns across populations? These questions are important because of the greater feasibility of the column-first approach (along with its greater susceptibility to the ecological fallacy).

The outstanding example of quantifying ill health is the Global Burden of Disease project (Murray and Lopez, 1996b), a tour de force of data assembly and summarization. Among its strong points are its explicit ethical foundation and its development of DALYs (see Section 2.2) as a population health index.

Interpreting Population Health Data

Rosén et al. (1985) provide guidelines for analyzing regional (mortality) data, suggesting that after a health problem has been chosen for analysis, the following "tests" be applied to the data:

1. Strength of the association with determinants (where relevant)
2. The regional pattern—are there consistent patterns?
3. Data quality
4. Consistency with other health indicators
5. Consistency with risk factors
6. Trend analysis
7. Consistency with other independent studies and with experiences of local health personnel.

Presenting the Health Status Profile

As with a meal, the presentation of a population health status profile is as critical as its content. Methods should be described, and their limitations discussed. Users appreciate presentation of data as graphs or maps, although these are easily overinterpreted. Tables have the advantage of being able to present data for several areas, along with summary data for the entire region or country; a case can be made for including such detailed data as appendices. It is tempting to include results that are not precise, both to avoid gaps and because these (often unexpected) results are often of most interest to readers, but this temptation should be avoided. It is important to include a considerable amount of discussion to guide readers who are not familiar with health issues; indeed, this is an essential part of the conversion of health information into health intelligence.

Small-Group Estimation

Planners and policymakers often need information about the health and risk factor status of small populations, defined geographically (e.g., residents of a neighborhood) or otherwise (e.g., members of occupational or ethnic groups). Local authorities are particularly interested in small populations, but the results upon which they try to base policy are often easily explained by chance alone. Health surveys rarely have a sufficiently large sample size to yield stable direct estimates for small populations. How should the epidemiologist proceed when faced with interesting but imprecise results? Confidence intervals are illuminating, albeit discouraging. The factors enumerated above by Rosén et al. help in interpreting small numbers. Any such interpretations should be regarded as highly tentative and subjected to early and frequent review, but a decision based on a cautious interpretation of weak data is usually sounder than one based on no data at all.

Several statistical techniques can be used to produce estimates of the prevalence of selected risk factors and health status indicators in small populations. These estimates are based on the selected population's sociodemographic characteristics (drawn from the census) and on the relation between these sociodemographic variables and the variables of interest (as shown by national or provincial health surveys) (Mackenzie et al., 1985). The assumption is that relation that hold at the national or provincial level also hold at the local level. In a similar vein, Rosén (1987:55) suggests that we use mortality data (which are available for small areas) to adjust national morbidity estimates to estimate morbidity in small areas. The main approaches are *synthetic estimation,* which is analogous to calculation of the expected numbers in indirect standardization, *multiple regression,* and combinations of the two. Synthetic estimation has not been found to be particularly promising because it captures only a small proportion of the variation and thus fails to reproduce the amount of dispersion that exists among small groups (Spasoff et al., 1996). Regression has been more successful, and a combination of the two approaches, including the synthetic estimate as an independent variable in a regression analysis, or using the difference between the synthetic estimate and the observed direct estimate as the dependent variable in a regression analysis, better yet, but the contribution of the approach remains limited (Purcell and Kish, 1979; Spasoff et al., 1996). Methodological advances in this area would be most useful. Box 4-2 describes a practical application.

Identifying Inequalities in Health

To a remarkable extent, wealth promotes health. The Black Report (Townsend and Davidson, 1992; Davey Smith et al., 1990) demonstrated that inequalities in health among social classes persisted several decades

---

Box 4-2. The Disease Impact Assessment System

Sainfort and Remington (1995) describe a spreadsheet program designed to produce estimates of the burden of several chronic diseases in a population. Essentially, it uses synthetic estimation, providing national age and sex-specific rates for incidence, prevalence, mortality and costs thereof, physician visits, hospital discharges and days, and direct health care costs for nine conditions. The user supplies population data for the target area and the program calculates the expected numbers for that population. Results in Wisconsin were fairly similar to the numbers observed in various state surveillance systems.

---

after introduction of the British National Health Service. Later, the Whitehall Study of British civil servants (Marmot et al., 1984) showed that the socioeconomic gradient in health existed across the entire job hierarchy, all of which was well above the poverty level. Caring people worry about this gradient. The health promotion movement attaches great importance to *equity* (fairness), based on the World Health Organization's (1981a) call for health for all, but this implies value judgements and is accordingly hard to conceptualize and measure. *Inequalities* in health among identifiable population groups are easier to measure and may or may not indicate the presence of inequity. Inequalities among socioeconomic groups are especially relevant to health policy and are the subject of most of the relevant research. The Black Report (Townsend and Davidson, 1992: 104 ff.) presented four hypotheses to explain such inequalities:

1. Artefact explanations, which arise problems in conceptualizing and measuring both health and class
2. Natural or social selection, or "health causing wealth," with downward social drift of the unhealthy
3. Materialist or structuralist explanations, which point to the role of material deprivation but go beyond it to suggest that an individual's position in society determines the opportunities available to the individual and thereby influences health
4. Cultural/behavioral explanations, which relate ill health to the unhealthful behaviors of low-income persons (ignoring the fact that the individual's position in society also determine the individual's choices among health-related behaviors) and perhaps to a "culture of poverty."

The Committee favored materialist/structuralist explanations, while acknowledging that the other hypotheses also play a role.

Methods to quantify inequalities in health have been borrowed from economics and studies of small-area variations in health care (Section 8.3), and epidemiologic methods have been adapted to the topic. Much more effort has been devoted to this topic in Europe than in North America, which has either clung to its myth of a classless society or substituted racial differences for class differences. Valuable reviews have been provided by Wagstaff et al. (1991) and Mackenbach and Kunst (1997). Ideally, such methods should incorporate independent or explanatory variables, especially socioeconomic status (SES), the example used here. They should reflect both the *effect* of the socioeconomic differences on individuals (shown by the RR) and the *impact* of such differences on the distribution of health in a population (dependent also on the distribution of SES across the population). When variables are dichotomous, inequalities in either health or its absence can be measured, and the results are not necessarily identical. Indicators of both absolute and relative differences among SES groups are needed because, like attributable risk and relative risk, these indicators have different policy implications. Available indicators can be considered under three headings, according to whether they show

1. inequalities among individuals or groups, with no independent variable (not discussed by Mackenbach and Kunst).
2. inequalities among groups defined by some explanatory variable, without regard to any pattern or gradient (Mackenbach and Kunst's "simple" measures).
3. inequalities among groups, the gradient being quantified by some explanatory variable (Mackenbach and Kunst's "sophisticated" measures).

Mackenbach and Kunst recommend using indicators of both effect on individuals and total impact on the population (two variants), and both absolute (difference) and relative (ratio) indicators. Inclusion of both simple and sophisticated variants of each leads to a total of 12 possible indicators, which are summarized in Table 4-2.

The indicators in the first group do not include any explanatory variables and thus merely show whether differences exist. The *Lorenz curve* is used by economists to illustrate the distribution of income or wealth across individuals and thus requires individual data. It is generated by arraying individuals in a population from least healthy to most healthy and then plotting the cumulative proportion of health against the cumulative proportion of individuals. The associated *Gini coefficient* is then the area between the Lorenz curve and the diagonal, as a proportion of the total area below the diagonal, and can vary from 0 to 1. In fact, the required individual data are often not available, but this is not catastrophic, since health differences among individuals are inevitable and not very

Table 4-2. A Systematic Overview of Possible Summary Measures of Health Inequality

Degree of Sophistication	Indices of Effect	Indices of Total Impact	
	Reference: High SES	Reference: High SES	Reference: Average SES
Simple	Rate difference	Population attributable risk	Index of dissimilarity (absolute)
	Rate ratio	Population attributable fraction	Index of dissimilarity (relative)
Sophisticated	Regression-based index of absolute effect	Regression-based population attributable risk	Slope index of inequality
	Regression-based index of relative effect	Regression-based population attributable fraction	Relative index of inequality

Reprinted from Social Science and Medicine 44, Mackenbach JP, Kunst, AE. Measuring the magnitude of socio-economic inequalities in health: an overview of available measures illustrated with two examples from Europe, pp.757–71, Copyright (1997), with permission from Elsevier Science.

interpretable; systematic differences among groups are much more important for health policy. Fortunately, relevant data are more often available for population groups; these data are the basis of several indicators. The *pseudo-Lorenz curve* and *pseudo-Gini coefficient* are calculated analogously to the individual versions by arraying the *groups* from least to most healthy, without regard to their SES (Wagstaff et al., 1991). Somewhat similar to the pseudo-Gini coefficient is the *Robin Hood index* (Kennedy et al., 1996), which divides the population into n health quantiles, selects those quantiles whose share of the total health exceeds $(100/n)\%$, and adds the excess of those shares above that level; it approximates the share of total health that would have to be taken from those above the mean and transferred to those below the mean to achieve equality in the distribution of health. It also equals the maximum vertical distance between the (pseudo-)Lorenz curve and the diagonal line of equal health. All of these indicators are of limited value because they fail to reveal any SES differences in health, although if the relationship between health and SES is monotonic, the pseudo-Lorenz curve and pseudo-Gini coefficient are identical to the concentration curve and index (see below), and do quantify such differences.

The simple indicators can detect differences among SES groups, but take no account of the pattern of these differences, e.g., of any gradient. The first two indicators, the *rate difference* and *rate ratio* (equivalent to the extremal quotient described in Section 8.3), use only the extreme groups, ignoring both the methods by which these groups have been defined and any patterns in the intervening majority of the population. The *population attributable risk* and *population attributable fraction* (see Section 2.3) treat (low) SES as a risk factor and use the highest SES group as the point of reference, which seems reasonable but does not work well if the relationship between health and SES is not monotonic. The *index of dissimilarity,* drawn from demography, is the number or proportion of cases (deaths, persons in a particular health category) whose health status category would have to change to eliminate health inequalities in the population (this number is usually divided by two to eliminate double counting). Wagstaff et al. and Mackenbach and Kunst offer different formulas, which are algebraically identical:

Index of Dissimilarity (Wagstaff)

$$= \frac{1}{2} \sum | p_{\text{health}} - p_{\text{population}} |$$

Index of Dissimilarity (Mackenbach and Kunst)

$$= \frac{1}{2N} \sum | n_{\text{equal}} - n_{\text{actual}} |$$

where p is the proportion of cases and of the population in each SES group, n_{equal} is the number of cases that would occur in each SES group if disease occurred at the same rate in each group, and N is the total number of cases. The index of dissimilarity equals half the population attributable fraction, except that its reference point is the average in the whole population rather than the lowest risk group. Since none of these approaches recognizes any possible gradient of health by SES, they would yield the same result if the categories were rearranged, even to the point of reversing the gradient.

The sophisticated indicators use regression analyses of the relation between SES and risk, and thus consider the gradient of risk. They reflect both the distribution of the population across SES groups and the relation between SES and health. The four "regression-based statistics" estimate the average health status of the groups from the regression of risk on SES, which should be measured by an interval variable; Wagstaff et al. (1991) note that because these are grouped data, weighted least squares should properly be used for this regression, rather than ordinary least squares. When the relation is clearly not linear, an appropriate transformation is indicated. Once the number of cases in each SES group has been predicted from the regression analysis, the calculation of the indicators parallels the simple indicators. The indices of inequality are based on the regression of the observed rates of disease in each SES group on the proportion of the population with lower income than the group's midpoint. The (generally negative) slope of this line is the *slope index of inequality*, and the ratio of the predicted probability of ill health for the least advantaged individual to that for the most advantaged individual is the *relative index of inequality* (as calculated by Mackenbach and Kunst).

The *concentration curve* and *concentration index* are similar to the pseudo-Lorenz and pseudo-Gini index, but array the groups by SES; they can accordingly show SES gradients. Wagstaff et al. conclude that the indices of inequality and the concentration index are the most useful indicators of inequalities in health and demonstrate their close mathematical relationship. Mackenbach and Kunst do not use the concentration index, partly because of that close relationship.

An example of the calculation of these indicators is found in Box 4-3. Of course, results for a single health indicator in a single jurisdiction are not very exciting; the results come to life when compared with other health indicators or other areas.

Economic Burden of Ill Health

The economic burden of ill health is the total economic cost of ill health to society, including both direct (costs of health care) and indirect costs (results of the ill health). Knowledge of the total economic burden of ill health is relevant to determining the appropriate amount of funding for health research and perhaps for health services. The breakdown of the total by diagnostic categories is relevant to allocating such funding: presumably the amount we spend on research for various disease categories should bear some relationship to the economic burden imposed by each. The measurements also have an integrating function in that they try to bring all the health effects into a single metric, in this case, dollars (cf. composite health indicators, Section 2.2). But there are also problems with this method. Disease-oriented foundations and drug companies have discovered the potential of emphasizing the importance of the diseases they address, and may be tempted to exaggerate the costs of those diseases. Some people object on principle to the concept of placing a dollar value on life and health, as required in estimating indirect burden.

Estimating the economic burden of ill health involves two steps: (1) measuring the amount of ill health (this is similar to preparation of a health profile, discussed above); and (2) assigning costs to the ill health. This section addresses the second step.

Direct costs are the costs of health care. Depending upon a jurisdiction's health information system, these may be fairly easy or very difficult to measure (see Section 3.4). There are problems in identifying diagnoses, especially in primary care, and in dealing with multiple diagnoses, which

Box 4-3. Identifying inequalities in health

Data from the Canadian National Population Health Survey of 1992 allow one to examine the relation between self-rated health and income adequacy. The results for Canadians aged 25–64 are shown in Box Table 4-3-1, and permit calculation of the recommended indicators.

Indicators of Inequalities in Self-rated Health, by Income Adequacy
Simple indicators

Rate difference = exposed attributable risk =
0.226 – 0.041 = 0.185 or 18% points

Rate ratio = extremal quotient = 0.226/0.041 = 5.5

Population attributable risk = 0.099 – 0.041 = 0.058 or 5.8% points

Population attributable fraction = (0.099 – 0.041)/0.099 = 0.59 or 59%

Index of dissimilarity (absolute) = 624,262/2 = 312,131 people

Index of dissimilarity (relative) =
(624,262/1)/14,337,697 = 0.022 or 2.2% (Kunst and Mackenbach)
or 0.044/2 = 0.022 or 2.2% (Wagstaff et al.)

Sophisticated indicators

Regressing the prevalence of fair or poor health on income adequacy (somewhat unforgivably coded 1 to 5) yields regression 1:
prevalence (F/P) = 0.269 – 0.0474 (income adequacy)

Regression-based index of absolute effect =
0.222 – 0.032 = 0.19 or 19% points

Regression-based index of relative effect = 0.222/0.032 = 6.8

Regression-based population attributable risk =
0.099 – 0.032 = 0.067 or 6.7 % points

Regression-based population attributable fraction =
(.099 – .032)/.099 = 0.68 or 68%

Regressing the prevalence of fair or poor health on the proportion of the population with lower income adequacy (and using ordinary least-squares regression) yields regression 2: prevalence (F/P) = 0.204 – 0.194 (proportion of population with lower income adequacy)

Slope index of inequality = -0.19

Relative index of inequality = (0.204 – 0.194 × 0)/(0.204 – 0.194 × 1) =
0.204/0.010 = 20

Other indicators
Pseudo-Lorenz curve: see Box Figure 4-3-1.
Pseudo-Gini coefficient (by geometry) = 0.015. Since the relationship between income adequacy and health is monotonic in this case, the concentration index is also 0.015.

(*continued*)

Box Table 4-3-1 Distribution of health by income adequacy

| | Income Adequacy | | | | |
Low	Lower	Middle	Upper	High (Reference)	Total
		Population (n pop)			
832,358	1,677,269	4,443,975	6,184,188	2,777,020	15,914,810
		Proportion of population (p pop)			
0.052	0.105	0.279	0.389	0.175	1.000
		Cumulative proportion			
0.052	0.157	0.436	0.825	1.000	
		Number E/VG/G (n "health")			
644,054	1,377,567	3,930,768	5,723,195	2,662,195	14,337,697
		Proportion E/VG/G (p health)			
0.045	0.096	0.274	0.399	0.186	1.000
		Cumulative proportion			
0.045	0.141	0.415	0.814	1.000	
		Number F/P health (n "sick")			
188,304	299,702	513,207	460,993	114,907	1,577,113
		Proportion sick (p sick)			
0.119	0.190	0.325	0.292	0.073	1.000
		Prevalence of sick (p)			
0.226	0.179	0.116	0.075	0.041	0.099
		RR for sick			
5.47	4.32	2.79	1.80	1.00	2.39
		pRR			
0.286	0.455	0.779	0.700	0.174	2.39
		Difference |p pop - p health|			
0.007	0.009	0.005	0.011	0.011	0.044
		Number sick if equal prevalence			
82,484	166,213	440,385	612,836	275,195	1,577,113
		Difference |n sick - n equal|			
105,820	133,489	72,822	151,843	160,288	624,262
		Code			
1	2	3	4	5	
		Predicted p sick (Regr 1)			
0.222	0.175	0.127	0.080	0.032	(0.099)
		RR for sick			
6.83	5.37	3.92	2.46	1.00	(continued)

Box Table 4-3-1 (*continued*)

Low	Lower	Middle	Upper	High (Reference)	Total
		Income Adequacy			
		RR for sick			
6.83	5.37	3.92	2.46	1.00	
		pRR			
0.357	0.566	1.094	0.955	0.175	3.15
		Population < midpoint			
416,179	1,670,993	4,731,615	10,045,696	14,526,300	
		Proportion < midpoint			
	0.026	0.105	0.297	0.631	0.913
		Predicted p sick (Regr2)*			
	0.204				0.010

*Estimated for the poorest and richest *individuals* in the population.

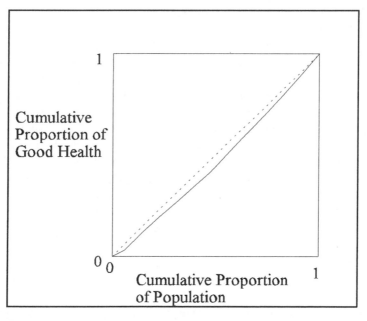

Box Figure 4-3-1. Pseudo-Lorenz Curve for distribution of excellent, very good, and good health among Canadians aged 25–64 years, as revealed by the 1992 National Population Health Survey. The population was divided into five categories of income adequacy, and then arrayed in order of increasing prevalence of good health. The dotted diagonal line represents equal distribution of health among categories, and the area between the diagonal line and the solid line, expressed as a proportion of the total area below the diagonal line, is the pseudo-Gini coefficient (here 0.015). Because the association between health and income adequacy is monotonic in this case, the pseudo-Lorenz curve and the pseudo-Gini coefficient equal the concentration curve and the concentration index.

are especially common in older people. Assigning the costs of drugs to disease categories is yet more difficult, since there is usually no source of administrative data and using consumption data is difficult because many drugs are used for more than one diagnosis. The whole costing process is usually dependent upon the prices of the various health services, which are often arbitrary and do not reflect the actual resource consumption. As with any economic analysis, there is the issue of the perspective from which the costs will be measured; for the purposes of policymaking, this should almost always be the perspective of society, and thus all costs should be included, regardless of who incurs or pays for them.

Indirect costs of ill health have two origins: morbidity and premature mortality. There are at least two approaches to this much more difficult costing process, which necessitates attaching a value to human life. The *human capital* approach, popularized by Rice (1966) in the United States equates the economic burden of morbidity or premature mortality to the resulting lost economic productivity, estimated by the present and future earnings that an individual would have made in the marketplace. This approach begins with the average earnings of people in a patient's age–sex group, and adjusts them for labor force participation, unemployment, etc. Future earnings are estimated from life expectancy and discounted to their present value. There are problems in using this approach to estimate the cost of ill health in women, for the method perpetuates the injustice of their low pay; homemakers and elders, whose market value is uncertain; and children, who lack earnings and for whom the choice of discount rate is critical. Especially in a time of high unemployment, sick or deceased workers may be rather quickly replaced, so the lost productivity to society may be less than that estimated by this approach. This approach also has no way of assigning costs to pain and suffering. Despite these criticisms, this approach is by far the most widely used.

The *willingness-to-pay* approach equates the burden imposed by a disease to the amount that people would pay to avoid having the disease. But which people should be studied: those who have the disease, or the general population? rich people or poor people? Economists are virtually unanimous in favoring this approach, but they appear to have failed to convince anyone else.

The *compensation and awards* approach has been proposed but perhaps never implemented. It bases its estimates of the economic burden imposed by a disease on the amounts awarded by courts, workers' compensation boards, etc. to people suffering from similar conditions in the belief that these amounts reflect the values that society places on avoiding the disease. But there may be no compensable "similar conditions," and the amounts of such awards may relate mainly to the skills of a lawyer or to the power or prestige of various groups in society.

Box 4-4 summarizes a recent study of the economic burden of illness.

Box 4-4. Economic burden of illness

A 1997 report (Moore et al., 1997) on the economic burden of ill health in Canada found that the total burden amounted to approximately U.S.$3,700 per capita per year. Direct costs comprised 46% and indirect costs 54% of the total. A major limitation was that about 38% of the direct costs (capital costs, some research costs, etc.) could not be allocated to diagnostic categories. For those costs that could be allocated, the leading disease categories were as follows:

Direct Costs	Indirect Costs	Total Costs
Cardiovascular 17%	Musculoskeletal 18%	Cardiovascular 15%
Mental 11%	Cardiovascular 14%	Musculoskeletal 14%
Respiratory 9%	Injuries 13%	Injuries 11%

The differences in rankings between direct and indirect costs are obvious. But the discrepancies between economic burden and research funding were even more obvious: the ratio of research funding to total disease burden varied by a factor of almost 50, from injuries at the low end to blood diseases at the high end. Other factors should influence research funding, but perhaps economic burden should play a greater role than it was playing in Canada.

Given the methodological difficulties in measuring this, a case can be made for expressing the indirect burden of ill health in terms of QALYs or DALYs lost, as was done in the Global Burden of Disease project (Murray and Lopez, 1996b), without attempting to express it in monetary terms. Admittedly, the result could not be added to direct burden to estimate the overall burden of ill health.

4.2 Assessing Health Needs

Purpose

Assessment of population health needs is necessary for policy development, health services planning, and resource allocation. The first problem is defining need.

Health Need, Want, and Demand

The definition of need has received much attention from health policy researchers, but nowhere near enough attention from practitioners. The *Dictionary of Epidemiology* (Last, 1995:111) offers a lengthy definition for health needs:

(Syn: health needs, perceived needs, professionally defined needs, unmet needs). This term has both a precise and an all-but-undefinable meaning in the context of public health. We speak of needs in precise numerical terms when we refer to specific indicators of disease or premature death that require intervention because their level is above that generally accepted in the society or community in question. For example, an infant mortality rate two or three times greater than the national average in a particular community is an indicator of unmet health needs of infants in that community (not to be confused with a need for more or better medical care). It should be clear that even in this seemingly precise usage, there are implied value judgments. It must be explicitly stated that "needs" always reflect prevailing value judgments as well as the existing ability to control a particular public health problem. Thus, sputum-positive pulmonary tuberculosis was not recognized as a health need in 1850 but was by 1900 in the industrialized nations; the ill effects of cigarette smoking must now be universally acknowledged as a health need; and child abuse is increasingly regarded as a public health problem to which we would apply the term professionally defined need.

The *Dictionary* then refers to Vickers's (1958) famous characterization of public health as "successive redefinings of the unacceptable," with its implications of societal expectations and technical possibilities. The definition suggests, and the public would certainly agree, that we cannot ignore standards of public service when defining need. But the definition is not easy to use in practice. Culyer's (1992:14) formulation has been adopted by many authorities, including the British National Health Service, and will be used here: "[N]eed is the minimum amount of resources needed to exhaust an individual's capacity to benefit." This conceptualization ties need to interventions: there is no such thing as a generalized need, only a need for some sort of intervention, which will often (but by no means always) be for health care. Furthermore, it implies that there can be need only for effective services, so needs assessment involves weighing evidence for effectiveness. "To speak of a need is to imply a goal, a measurable deficiency from the goal, and a means of achieving the goal" (Wilkin et al., 1992:2). Culyer refers not to capacity to benefit but to the resources needed to exhaust the capacity to benefit although most users ignore this distinction. The reference to resources suggests that we should also consider the costs of the interventions and address the ability of some people to benefit more than others from a given expenditure. The concept of *avoidable mortality,* introduced by Rutstein et al. (1976) as a tool for measuring quality of care, seems useful in understanding and measuring need. They identified a number of conditions (e.g., ruptured appendix) that should not happen in a well-functioning health-care system and argued that any occurrence of such a condition indicates a deficiency in health care. Inasmuch as the mortality and morbidity could have been avoided by (better) health services, the persons suffering from them had the capacity to benefit from such interventions, and thus were in need. Others have since extended the concept to avoidable morbidity and disability.

Stevens and Raftery (1994:4) place the conceptualization of need in a broader context, quoting Bradshaw's distinction among four approaches to defining social need:

- *normative* need, defined "objectively" by professionals;
- *felt* need, defined "subjectively" by the individual, and equivalent to want or expectation;
- *expressed* need, as indicated by people's actions, e.g., in seeking care; this need is related to demand, the amount of services that an individual would utilize at a given cost, and effective demand or utilization;
- *comparative* need, which is a lower use of services than enjoyed by some comparable population.

A fifth operational definition may be added, drawn from lay usage: existence of a health problem.

None of these concepts considers the effectiveness or even the existence of potential interventions. Defining need as health problems identifies limitless amounts of need, while using someone else's utilization as an estimate of need can lead to gross inefficiencies.

Yet another distinction is needed. It is important to distinguish between *met* and *unmet* needs, according to whether people are receiving effective services. One could argue that a met need is no longer a need, and that needs are by definition unmet, but in practice it is useful to retain both concepts. Obviously, met need is related both to demand and supply, and unmet need is of special interest to the policymaker.

Identifying Health Needs at the Population Level

According to Pickin and St Leger (1993), "[h]ealth needs assessment is the process of exploring the relationship between health problems in a community and the resources available to address these problems in order to achieve a desired outcome." Wright et al. (1998:1310) expand the definition to include efficiency: "Health needs assessment is the systematic approach to ensuring that the health service uses its resources to improve the health of the population in the most efficient way." Defining the needs of an individual in a clinical situation is quite different from defining the needs of a population, the problem confronting the policy epidemiologist: the clinician usually does not (and perhaps should not) worry about costs, but the policymaker must. Conducting a needs assessment is more than preparing a health profile; need implies the existence of an effective intervention and the possibility of providing it, whereas measuring health status need not consider these factors.

The epidemiological approach to health care needs assessment (Stevens and Raftery, 1994), developed in the United Kingdom, is a comprehensive approach to population needs assessment; not surprisingly, it is the most appealing approach for an epidemiologist. Two large volumes have been published, presenting application of the method to a large number of diseases. Despite its title, this approach is both epidemiologically and economically based. The authors contrast it with the *comparative* approach, which contrast the services received in the population in one area with those received by other populations, in its avoidance of using utilization as a measure of need, and the *corporate* approach, which canvasses the demands, wishes, and alternative perspectives of professionals, politicians, the public, and other interested parties, in its use of objective measures (Stevens and Raftery, 1994:10–12). Stevens and Raftery list the purposes of needs assessment as support for purchasing services (a crucial issue in the British National Health Service), resource allocation, and attempts to enhance efficiency, or ensuring that services are getting to the right people. They reduce Culyer's definition of need to the population's ability to benefit from health care, noting that the service must be effective on average, and that health care is broadly defined to include patient and caregiver support. Three types of information are considered; these are illustrated in Figure 4-1 as the corners of a triangle. The model comprises the following steps:

1. Statement of the context of the problem (usually best defined in terms of diseases, not populations or services)
2. Formation of subcategories for analysis (usually functional, in terms of disability, not anatomic or pathological)

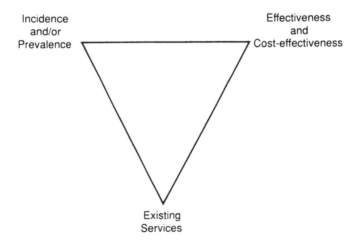

Figure 4-1. The triangulation of health care needs assessment.
Source: Stevens and Raftery (1994:6), with permission.

3. Estimation of prevalence and/or incidence of the disease. For acute problems, incidence is the most useful indicator. For chronic problems, prevalence is most useful for continuing care, but incidence identifies the need for services provided once per case, e.g., the initial management of a condition
4. Estimation of current service provision
5. Assessment of effectiveness and cost-effectiveness of services, using an approach based on that of the Canadian Task Force on the Periodic Health Examination (1994) and the U.S. Preventive Services Task Force (1996) to evaluate evidence
6. Definition of models of care. Conceding that a simple formula will rarely be adequate, Stevens and Raftery suggest that services be categorized simultaneously by subcategory and service level and that a model of care be defined by the priority (high, medium, low, or nil) assigned to each cell (see Table 4-3).
7. Specification of outcomes and targets (including needed research and information).

The life cycle framework of Pickin and St. Leger (1993) also comprises three activities: health status measurement, identification of ways of maximizing health gain, and measurement of health resources (equivalent to the triangle of Stevens and Raftery). They see a community as a small geographical area with an upper-limit population of 12,000 and recommend use of a life-cycle framework with nine age-groups over the traditional approaches based on types of services or client groups. In contrast to the epidemiologic approach, they suggest an important role for qualitative research including observation, informal interviewing, group interviewing, focus groups, document analysis. They note that rapid appraisal can gain insight into a community's own perspective on priority needs, help to translate these findings into managerial action, and establish an on-going relationship between funders, providers and local communities (cf. rapid epidemiologic assessment [Smith, 1989]). The process is carried out in four steps:

Table 4-3. Definition of Model of Care, with Sample Priorities

Subcategory	Service Level		
	Prevention	Treatment	Rehabilitation
Population at large	High	Nil	Nil
Mild disease	Medium	Medium	Low
Severe disease	Low	Medium	High

Source: Stevens and Raftery (1994:16), with permission.

1. Identify pertinent life cycle stages.
2. Quantify the extent of the health needs and problems within each stage.
3. Apply health modifiers (socioeconomic, environmental, ethnic, cultural) to each stage.
4. Relate the health status progression in steps 1–3 to health resources.

Chambers et al. (1983) present a less structured approach to needs assessment in which the following major questions are addressed:

1. Can the reasons for proposing a particular need be identified?
2. Can the health need be reduced or alleviated?
3. What factors will influence decision makers to maintain, add to, or decrease current efforts to meet this health need?
4. Are improvements or changes required?
5. Should a new program be implemented; should current programs be maintained, changed, curtailed; or should servicing of this perceived need be abandoned?

Chambers et al. identify available sources of information for each step.

Identifying unmet needs

It is difficult to put into practice the capacity to benefit at the population level, at least if the interest is in determining unmet need. The published methods are clear about assessing health problems and available resources but vague about bringing the two together (step 6 in the epidemiological approach, step 4 in the life cycle framework). Are the individuals in need receiving the appropriate interventions? In principle, linked morbidity and utilization data should permit the definition of unmet need. But there are at least three problems with this approach: (1) very few jurisdictions possess any such data; (2) it is difficult to imagine a population in which morbidity data are available for all individuals (except for utilization data, which have already been branded as unsuitable), although it should be possible to link health survey results to utilization data and generalize the result to the whole population; and (3) not all persons with a given health problem need a given intervention, even when that intervention has been shown to be effective for the condition. Other variables or factors such as comorbidity, contraindications, and availability of alternative treatment may determine whether an individual needs a service. Administrative data of this complexity will never be available. The following approach may help to differentiate between met and unmet needs:

1. Determine from the literature which interventions have been shown to be beneficial for each health problem.

2. Form problem-intervention pairs and proceed with one pair at a time, beginning with a blank table similar to Table 4-4 for each pair.
3. Determine the proportion of patients with the problem that can be expected to benefit from the intervention using a combination of evidence, consensus and standards, and thereby estimate the total need the total number of individuals who need the intervention; see right margin of Table 4-4).
4. Measure the actual level of utilization of the intervention by persons with the problem, i.e., the total number of individuals treated (bottom margin of Table 4-4). If only overall utilization is available, not utilization by persons with the problem in question, estimate the proportion and number of users who have the disease.
5. Assess the fit between need and provision of the intervention, i.e., attempt to fill in the cells of Table 4-4. If all persons with the disease need the intervention, then cells c and d are empty. If it can be reasonably assumed that the intervention is never provided to persons without the indication, then cell $c = 0$, and the remaining cells can be filled by subtraction. Otherwise, it may be possible to estimate from the literature or expert judgement the proportion of persons with the disease who lack the indications for the intervention but still receive it, allowing cell c to be estimated and the remaining cells to be filled by subtraction.
6. In the absence of any information regarding the cells, then more limited conclusions may be drawn from the numbers needing and receiving services:

- Number in Need > Number Treated: at least some unmet need exists
- Number in Need = Number Treated: compatible with equal offsetting deficiencies (cell b = cell c)
- Number in Need < Number Treated: at least some unnecessary care is being provided.

Table 4-4. Measuring Need (applies to a specific problem-intervention pair)

	Receiving Intervention	Not Receiving Intervention	Total
Intervention is indicated	(*a*) Met need	(*b*) Unmet need	Total need for intervention
Intervention is not indicated	(*c*) Inappropriate treatment	(*d*) Appropriate non-treatment	No need for intervention
TOTAL	Total treated	Not treated	Total cases of problem

The possibility of offsetting errors limits interpretability of the results, since the people in need may not be those receiving the intervention (an example of the ecological fallacy).

Data Sources for Needs Assessment

Many of the data sources listed for inclusion in a population health information system are relevant (Section 3.4). In addition, there will usually be a need for specially collected data, which may take several forms.

Quantitative data

There may be a case for conducting a health survey in the population, given the usual inadequacy of sample sizes from national surveys. There is a tendency for politicians and other community representatives to respond much more positively to data that originate in their own communities, so even a little local information may strengthen a case considerably. But a health survey is very expensive and the sample size will still prove inadequate to support many breakdowns. An unfortunate feature of surveys is that the sample size required for the desired degree of precision is needed for each subgroup that may be of interest. Small-area estimation (see Section 4.1) may eventually solve this problem, as techniques improve. Surveys of local health professionals and agencies should be considered, but in general are not population based and so do not necessarily convey an accurate picture of the needs of the whole population; furthermore, the picture they convey is filtered through professional eyes and ears.

Capture–recapture (capture-mark-recapture) methods These methods can improve the completeness of estimates of disease occurrence, especially for conditions like drug addiction and mental illness, for which most data sources are weak. Originally developed in biology as the basis of bird-banding programs, these methods are based on ascertaining the occurrence of disease from at least two sources. The simple situation can be summarized in a 2×2 table:

	Source B	
	Detected	Not detected
Source A		
Detected	a	b
Not detected	c	

Provided that the sources of ascertainment are independent (which is admittedly rarely the case), then the total number of cases in the population is estimated by the reverse of the process for computing an expected value in a contingency table (Hook and Regal, 1992):

$$\text{Maximum Likelihood Estimate (MLE)} = \frac{(a + b)\,(a + c)}{a}$$

$$\text{Nearly Unbiased Estimate (NUE)} = \frac{(a + b + 1)\,(a + c + 1)}{a + 1} - 1$$

where a is the number identified by both sources and b and c are the numbers identified by one source, but not the other. If more than two sources are available, then the assumption of independence can be tested. The variance of the NUE is (Laporte et al., 1992):

$$\text{Variance (NUE)} = \frac{(a + b + 1)\,(a + c + 1)\,(b)\,(c)}{(a + 1)^2\,(a + 2)}$$

Box 4-5 provides a simple example. By applying the capture–recapture method, Hook and Regal (1992) found that their prevalence survey had missed 25%–40% of the cases of Huntingdon's disease in a community;

Box 4-5. Capture–Recapture Methods

Laporte et al. (1992) illustrated the method with Swedish data on the occurrence of myocardial infarction (MI), drawn from the Monitoring Cardiovascular Disease (MONICA) project. During a certain period of time, the MI registry registered 5832 cases and the hospital discharge index registered 6582; of these, 4746 were captured by both sources. These data are presented below in a 2 × 2 table.

	Hospital Discharges		
MI Registry	Yes	No	Total
Yes	4746	1086	5832
No	1836		
Total	6582		

The maximum likelihood estimate (MLE) of the total cases in the population is then (5832 × 6582)/4746 = 8088 and the nearly unbiased estimate (NUE) is also {(5833 × 6583)/4747} – 1 = 8088.

The variance of the latter is (5833)(6583)(1086)(1836)/{(4747²)(4748)} = 716, leading to a 95% confidence interval of 8088 ± 1.96 √716 = 8036, 8140.

The MI registry identified 5832/8088 = 72% of the estimated total cases, whereas the hospital system identified 6582/8088 = 81%. Both sources together identified (5832 + 6582 – 4746)/8088 = 95% of cases.

they accordingly recommend that "no attempted completed prevalence studies be presented without data on ascertainment by source intersection," and even suggest that capture–recapture may produce a new paradigm for human population science: we age-adjust, so why do we not also ascertainment-adjust? An International Working Group for Disease Monitoring and Forecasting (1995) agrees, but other authors are less sanguine about the contribution of the approach (Desenclos and Hubert, 1994; Papoz et al., 1996).

Qualitative data

Qualitative methods can make a key contribution to a needs assessment by helping to explain why things are happening, and the intense pictures that they provide can give life to a rigorous but gray statistical report. Methods include the use of focus groups and of key informants such as community leaders and health professionals. A detailed description is available in Morse and Field (1995).

4.3 Risk and Risk Assessment

While needs assessment refers to the possibility of providing services to a population, risk assessment refers to hazards to which they are exposed.

Risk

The word "risk" has many and changing uses. In modern epidemiology it refers to cumulative incidence, which is the probability that an individual will develop a certain outcome within a certain time. After providing a similar definition, the *Dictionary of Epidemiology* (Last, 1995:148) adds that risk is "[a]lso, a nontechnical term encompassing a variety of measures of the probability of a (generally) unfavorable outcome." Another common use is the probability of an event multiplied by its consequences.

Risk Perception

Much is known about the way that individuals perceive and assess risk, especially their difficulty in understanding probability. In general, rare outcomes, especially disasters, are assessed as more probable than they actually are, whereas common outcomes, especially if they result from voluntary exposures, are assessed as less probable than they actually are. Similarly, people are more accepting of self-induced risks than of those that are imposed upon them.

Risk Assessment

Environmental risk assessment

This well-developed discipline belongs in this book because it concerns situations in which governments make policy and to which epidemiology can contribute (Samet and Burke, 1998). Environmental risk assessment developed as a means of helping governments decide what to do about environmental hazards like nuclear wastes and PCBs, but the principles apply equally to hazardous effects of drugs or medical treatments. Thus, it brings epidemiologists into contact with toxicologists, who have adduced much of the evidence in this field, mainly through animal experimentation and mainly regarding carcinogens. In toxicology, high exposure levels can be studied under more controlled conditions, but epidemiology has greater external validity, given its focus on free-standing human populations. Hertz-Picciotto (1995) argues that risk assessment provides a bridge between science and policy and proposes a classification framework for assessing the contribution of individual epidemiologic studies to that process. In the United States, the National Research Council (1983) identified four components of the risk assessment process, in an approach that has become standard.

1. Hazard identification. What is the hazard or exposure, and what adverse health effects does it produce? This evaluation is based on laboratory toxicological research, descriptive epidemiology, especially ecological studies, and analogy, among others.

2. Hazard assessment (dose–response assessment). This particularly difficult step tries to determine the shape of the dose–response curve. Is there a threshold, or is there no completely safe level of exposure? Figure 4-2

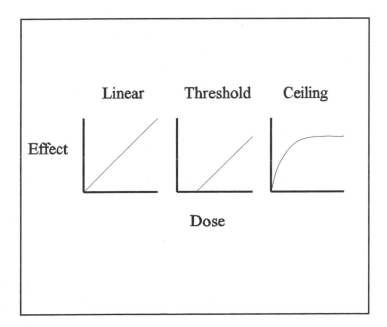

Figure 4-2. Dose-response patterns. In the linear pattern, any exposure is harmful, and risk rises proportionally with dose. In the threshold pattern there is no effect below a certain level of exposure, but risk rises proportionally with dose above that level. In the ceiling pattern, risk rises proportionally with dose, but levels off at a certain point. Many combinations and other patterns are possible.

shows three patterns. Laboratory studies normally use far higher doses than those to which humans are ever exposed, and even epidemiologic studies tend to use highly exposed populations (e.g., occupational groups) to observe a sufficient number of events without studying immense numbers of individuals. The challenge is to extrapolate these results to the low exposure levels to which the bulk of the population is exposed, as exemplified by the attempts to assess the safety of low-dose radiation.

3. Exposure assessment. A hazard will not damage health unless people are exposed to it—indeed, unless their vulnerable target organs are exposed to it. In environmental risk assessment, this step involves quantifying the emissions of a pollutant into the environment, its ambient levels in the environment, levels of human exposure, the amount entering humans, and finally, the dose of the substance which reaches the vulnerable organs. The effective exposure (at the tissue level) is highly dependent upon individual behaviors and habits as well as individual biology. At the level of populations, exposure assessment involves estimating the number of persons who are exposed to a certain drug or procedure or who will engage in a certain behavior.

4. Risk characterization. This quantitative step relates the expected exposure (step 3) to the expected outcomes (step 2). Often it involves using a mathematical model to calculate the expected numbers of cases or deaths in a particular situation, as attempted in disease modeling (Section 6.2). The key statistic is population attributable risk, the absolute number of cases of attributable to the exposure (see Section 2.3).

Behavioral risk assessment

Unlike environmental risk assessment, this is normally carried out at the level of individuals, since behaviors are individual. It is relevant here because the determinants of health behavior often act at the population level. *Health risk appraisal* (HRA) is a health education tool that uses information on an individual's personal (mostly behavioral) risk factors to estimate the probability that the individual will die during the next 10 years, in the belief that this knowledge will help to motivate individuals to change their health behaviors (DeFriese, 1987). In the 1980s the development of HRA was supported by the governments of both the United States ("Healthier People") and Canada ("Evalu-Life"). Its population equivalent, Prevent, is addressed in Box 6-6. As originally developed, HRA uses population mortality rates for each age–sex group to estimate the corresponding (average) probabilities of death over the next 10 years, overall, from each of the 12 leading causes of death, which usually account for about 70% of all deaths, and from all other causes combined. To appraise an individual's risk of death from a specific disease, the probability in the population is multiplied by a factor that reflects the individual's risk factors:

$$\text{Individual Multiplier} = \frac{RR_i}{\Sigma pRR}$$

where the RR_i is the relative risk associated with the individual's level of exposure, p is the prevalence of each level of exposure, and ΣpRR is the average relative risk in the population. Thus, it is a sort of relative risk in which the reference is the risk associated with the average exposure rather than the risk in the unexposed. The multiplier is assigned a value of 1 for diseases for which no risk factors have been determined, including diseases ranking below 12th in mortality. The individual's probabilities of death from each disease are added to produce an overall *appraised probability of death*. Exposure levels for modifiable risk factors are then changed to the least hazardous feasible level, and the whole process is repeated to generate an *achievable probability of death*. Complications arise when there is more than one risk factor for a condition, since the calculations must then reflect the causal model (additive, multiplicative, or other)—information that is rarely known (Spasoff and McDowell, 1987). The multiplier is closely related to the population attributable fraction (PAF; Section 2.3), and similar conditions for its validity and manipulation apply. As for the PAF, a valid approach is to combine all the exposures into a single composite variable; information on the joint distributions of the risk factors is needed and is usually the limiting factor for this approach. For ischemic heart disease and stroke, logistic regression equations that can replace the above procedure are available, although such models make strong assumptions and impose heavy data requirements. The model has been extended to appraise the risk of various types of morbidity, with all the methodological problems noted under disease modeling (Section 6.2). DeFriese and Fielding (1990) review opportunities and challenges for the future.

Risk Communication

As noted above, probabilities are hard to understand. Various metrics have been developed to help people understand levels of risk, e.g., that a certain exposure has the same risk as crossing the street, but these comparisons are often simplistic. In health risk appraisal, the appraised and achievable probabilities of death are converted to equivalent ages, or the age at which the average individual has the same risk as the person whose risk is being appraised. This conversion improves comprehension but encounters problems when the risk of death does not rise monotonically with age, as is often found in young men: there can then be three or more equivalent ages for a single level of risk.

Risk Management

This area concerns subsequent policy interventions (e.g., regulations, education, taxes) or lack thereof. In the case of environmental exposures, people tend to demand that their level of risk be zero, but this is obviously not possible. The acceptable exposure may be derived from the level at which no observable adverse effect is observed (NOAEL). When (as is usually the case) the model is based on animal data, there arises the question of extrapolating the results to humans. It is common to introduce a safety factor, often a tenfold decrease, in the dose to which people may be exposed, and then a similar factor to account for variation among humans in their sensitivity to the agent. Many health promotion policies address behavioral risks at the population level (e.g., community development, tobacco policies, educational programs).

4.4 Assessing Causes of Health Problems

After the health problems afflicting a population have been identified and quantified, it is necessary to consider their causes, with a view to preventing the problems. There is no need to treat etiologic research in general here, since most epidemiologic textbooks have that focus. An exception is *ecological studies,* which are demeaned in mainstream epidemiology but deserve a higher rating for policy purposes. The epidemiologist working on policy needs to be able to *assess* the etiologic research done by others for relevance to policy issues.

Contribution of Ecological Studies

Ecological (correlational) *studies* are studies in which the unit of observation and analysis is the group, not the individual. These studies are attractive because of their convenience and low cost: the necessary data are often readily available in published reports. A much more important advantage is that many determinants of health operate at the population level, as do many of the interventions at the disposal of policymakers, such as advertising restrictions, environmental regulations, and influences on the social environment; paradoxically, epidemiology is defined as being concerned with the health of populations, but most epidemiologic studies are based on individuals and highest status is assigned to such studies. Epidemiologists working with policymakers will be asked to interpret the results of ecological studies and may be asked to undertake them. Excellent overviews of ecological studies have been provided by Morgenstern (1982, 1995) and Susser (1994).

Variables

Morgenstern (1995) notes that variables can be measured at various levels:

1. *Individual*: conventional microdata
2. *Aggregate*: summaries (means or proportions) of individual measurements, for example, average diastolic blood pressure or the proportion of people with body mass index >27
3. *Environmental*: characteristics measured at the group level for which there is an individual analogue; for example, ambient levels of air pollutants that could be measured with personal monitors to obtain individual exposure levels.
4. *Global*: attributes of groups or places for which there is no clear analogue at the individual level. Examples are population density or living under a particular form of government.

Designs and analysis
Morgenstern's (1995) most recent categorization of designs is presented in Table 4-5, with examples. *Analysis* may also be carried out at several different levels.

1. Individual level analysis. Each individual has a value for each variable, as in the typical analytical epidemiologic study. With population data, this level implies that the joint distributions of all combinations of variables are available.

2. Completely ecologic analysis. All variables are ecologic, and the unit of analysis is the group. The marginal distributions of all the variables are available, but not their joint distributions. In a multiple-group analytical study, the variables are continuous (means or proportions) and the appropriate analysis is regression. The ecological correlation coefficient can be estimated as follows (Morgenstern, 1982):

$$R_{ecol} = B_1 \sqrt{\frac{varx}{vary}}$$

where varx and vary are the variances of X and Y, and B_1 is the slope when Y is regressed on X. Similarly, the ecologic relative risk for a 1-unit increase in X is estimated by

$$RR_{ecol} = 1 + \frac{B_1}{B_0}$$

where B_0 is the regression constant (intercept). For time trends, *age-period-cohort analysis* is available for exploratory purposes (see Section 8.2) and *autoregressive integrated moving average* (ARIMA) models for analytical purposes; the latter assess the effects of independent variables and account for the lack of independence of the data from various years (Helfenstein, 1991).

Table 4-5. Ecological Study Designs, with Examples

Study Design	Exploratory (primary exposure not measured)	Analytic (primary exposure measured and analyzed)
Multiple-group (measured at a single time	Mortality atlas	Mortality rate by average income
Time-trend (for a single group)	Time trend of a disease in a population	Changes in smoking versus changes in cancer rates over time
Mixed study (multiple groups over time)	Time trends for several populations	As above, for several populations

Source: Data adapted from Morgenstern (1995).

3. Partially ecologic analysis. This analysis incorporates some but not all joint distributions of risk factors and outcomes.

4. Combined analyses. These analyses include both individual and group variables. In *contextual analysis,* the analysis is conducted at the individual level, with individuals in a group assigned the average values of the measured environmental and global variables for their groups. The results are subject to problems resulting from *intraclass correlation* (within-group clustering). *Multilevel analysis (hierarchical regression, random-effects modeling)* is a modeling technique that combines analyses at two or more levels. Multilevel models are complicated, but Hox (1995) presents a very clear conceptual introduction. A regression model containing all the independent variables believed to act at the level of the individual is applied separately within each grouping at the next higher level, so that a different set of coefficients is estimated for each group (i.e., the relations are not assumed to be identical in every group; cf. the random effects model in meta-analysis, Section 5.2). For a two-level model with only one variable at each level this is of the form:

$$Yij = \beta_0 j + \beta_1 jXij + eij$$

where Y and X refer to the ith individual of the jth group, X representing the independent variables believed to operate at the individual level. The regression coefficients become the dependent variables for the next higher level, with the independent variables being those believed to act at that level (here represented by Z). For the jth group, this is:

$$\beta_0 j = \gamma_{00} + \gamma_{01} Zj + u_0 j$$
$$\beta_1 j = \gamma_{10} + \gamma_{11} Zj + u_1 j$$

Inserting the latter values into the first equation yields

$$Yij = \gamma_{00} + \gamma_{01}Zj + u_0j + \gamma_{10}Xij + \gamma_{11}ZjXij + u_1jXij + eij$$
$$= \gamma_{00} + \gamma_{01}Zj + \gamma_{10}Xij + \gamma_{11}ZjXij + u_0j + u_1jXij + eij$$

The first four terms are the fixed (deterministic) portion of the equation, the fourth term represents cross-level interaction, and the last three terms are the random (stochastic) portion. Such analyses can require estimation of a remarkably large number of parameters. For example, with two levels of analysis (individuals and groups) and two explanatory variables at each level, there are 15 parameters, compared to only 6 when all the explanatory variables are considered to act a single level. The interpretation of some of these parameters can be quite subtle, but the approach is much needed and papers using it are beginning to appear in the epidemiologic literature (see Box 4-6). The analyses can be accomplished with standard statistical packages, although specialized computer programs are available.

Methodologic problems.
Ecologic studies are subject to several types of methodologic problems (Morgenstern, 1995):

1. *within-group bias,* in the several well-known varieties that also afflict individual-level studies;
2. *confounding by group* (peculiar to ecologic studies), in which the associations between variables are different within the various groups;
3. *effect modification by group* (also peculiar to ecologic studies), in which the true effects of a variable are different in different groups.

The last two categories can cause *cross-level bias,* a general term used to refer to a situation in which a relationship that holds at one level of aggregation is incorrectly assumed to hold at another level of aggregation. Both errors should be reduced by multilevel analysis. The older literature focused on the *ecological fallacy,* in which relations that apply at the group level do not apply at the individual level (which was assumed to represent the truth). More recent examinations emphasize that the "truth" depends upon the level at which variables exert their effect and take a more symmetrical position (Schwartz, 1994). Thus, cross-level bias may take the form of either an *ecological fallacy,* which is incorrectly assuming that aggregate results apply to individuals, or an *atomistic fallacy,* which is incorrectly assuming that individual results apply to groups. The bottom line is that we should conduct the analysis at whatever level makes sense for the particular variables at hand.

Box 4-6. Multilevel analysis

O'Campo et al. (1997) studied the determinants of low birthweight in Baltimore, considering both individual and neighborhood risk factors. The statistically significant results (odds ratios [OR] for direct effects, sign for direction of interaction effects) were as follows:

Individual Factors	OR	Neighborhood Factors	OR
Direct effects			
Maternal age	1.02	Average income <$8,000	1.11
Maternal education	0.87		
Late prenatal care	1.25		
Medicaid recipient	1.49		
Interaction effects, entering through:			
Maternal age		Unemployment rate	(+)
Maternal education		Crime rate	(−)
Late prenatal care		(Log) average wealth	(−)
		Unemployment rate	(−)
Medicaid recipient		Average income <$8000	(−)
		Average income $8000-11,000	(−)

The effects of several individual-level factors depended upon the characteristics of the neighborhood. For example, the adverse effects of being on Medicaid or starting prenatal care late were reduced in poorer areas. A high crime rate in the neighborhood reduced the protective effect of maternal education. High unemployment increased the already elevated risk in older women. The investigators concluded that design of programs directed at reducing the prevalence of low birthweight should consider neighborhood as well as individual risk factors.

Critical Appraisal of Etiological Studies

Epidemiologists possess the expertise needed to evaluate evidence and a tradition of critical evaluation of their own and others' work. Clinical epidemiologists in particular have developed critical appraisal of medical evidence to a high level. Since the clinician is usually more interested in what to do about the patient's problems than in what caused them, the resulting guides tend to discuss causation only in the context of adverse effects of treatments (Levine et al., 1994).

Internal validity

It is rarely possible to use randomized (or even nonrandomized intervention) designs in searching for the causes of health problems, so the available evidence comes mainly from observational studies. Some recalibration is therefore necessary when using the critical appraisal approaches developed for clinicians managing individual patients: a cohort design may be inexcusable when evaluating an intervention but is usually the best possible design when evaluating the effects of an exposure (Section 5.1). But the general principles used to assess internal validity in etiological and clinical epidemiology apply equally to epidemiology for health policy.

External validity

Policy development and evaluation often involve applying research results to other populations and other times. External validity is therefore a greater problem than in clinical medicine, since the social and health system factors contributing to health and disease in a specific population may be rather specific to that population and may not have been addressed in published research. Issues to consider include the following:

- demographic composition of the population, including age, sex, social structure, and education;
- political structure, including health and social services and income support;
- economic status, including level of wealth and its distribution;
- culture, including attitudes toward health and health-related behavior.

Summary

Measurement of health depends upon the definition adopted. Since we usually cannot measure health directly, we use indicators, which often measure the absence of health (e.g., mortality, morbidity). Indices combine two or more indicators into a larger construct; much work has been done on indices using microdata, but less has been done on indices using aggregated population health data. A population health profile can be useful for goal-setting or resource allocation. Use of administrative (routinely collected) data is attractive because of convenience and economy, but surveys are the only ways to obtain information on self-rated health or health beliefs or behaviors. Surveys rarely have the sample size needed to describe small populations; small-group estimation techniques show some promise for resolving this problem. Assessment of inequalities in health is important for development of health policy. Estimates of the economic burden of the ill health faced by a population can help to set priorities for health research and health services. Epidemiologists are often asked to assess the health needs of a population. Need is the resources required to exhaust the capacity of an individual to benefit from a health care intervention; there can therefore be need only for effective care. Needs assessment should be based on multiple sources of information, including the opinions of the population concerned and of key informants such as local health care providers. Risk assessment can refer to either environmental or individual (usually behavioral) risks. Eventual interventions will be based upon what is known about the etiology of the health problems. Ecological studies are often the most feasible; when variables act at the level of the group, they are also the most appropriate. Such studies are subject to cross-level bias, which can be avoided by appropriate use of variables and analytical techniques. Criteria developed in clinical settings to assess the potential of a study to yield valid information require recalibration for use in population settings. *External validity* is particularly important in assessing the value of etiological studies for policy development.

Key References

Health Needs Assessment [series of six articles]. *BMJ* 1998; 316.

Mackenbach JP, Kunst AE. Measuring the magnitude of socio-economic inequalities in health: an overview of available measures illustrated with two examples from Europe. *Soc Sci Med* 1997;44:757–71.

Morgenstern H. Ecologic studies in epidemiology: concepts, principles, and methods. *Annu Rev Public Health* 1995;16:61–81.

Samet JM, Burke TA. Epidemiology and risk assessment. In: Brownson RC, Petitti DB (eds). *Applied Epidemiology: Theory to Practice.* New York: Oxford University Press, 1998;137–75 .

5

Assessment of Potential Interventions

We shall distinguish here between interventions, or individual treatments or programs, and policies, or integrated packages including one or more interventions together with goals and implementation strategies. Assessment of an intervention involves several stages: assessment of individual evaluations of the intervention, synthesis of the relevant evidence, and assessment of the suitability of the intervention for health policy development. Only after each of the alternatives has been assessed in this way is it possible to make an informed decision on which one to implement, the topic of Chapter 6. This very complex topic is addressed by entire disciplines (health care technology assessment) and books (Muir Gray, 1997); this chapter provides an overview.

5.1 Assessing Evidence from Intervention Studies

The first step in assessing interventions for inclusion in health policy is assessment of the evidence arising from individual studies of interventions. The evidence base for evaluating the options is often weak, but just as the clinician must decide what to do for the patient, using the best available evidence, so the policymaker must make decisions, however weak the knowledge base. It is up to the epidemiologist to assess that knowledge base and make the best possible recommendations. Here we assume that at least some empirical evidence already exists in the form of research reports of evaluative studies. If no such evidence exists, then policymaking is premature and the first priority is to generate the basic evidence, which shifts the focus to clinical trials and health services research, which are beyond the scope of this book.

How do we identify the interventions to be assessed? Some will be presented by their proponents, but not necessarily the most promising ones! It is better to do a literature search and to consult experts and other jurisdictions to identify interventions that address the population's health problems. If faced with a flood of possibilities, it may be necessary to set some screening criteria, for instance, quality of available evidence and consistency with overall policy thrusts, to allow attention to be focussed on the more promising interventions.

Beginning with critical appraisal of the medical literature (Department of Clinical Epidemiology and Biostatistics, 1981; Sackett et al., 1991), epidemiologists have been concerned with evaluating the quality of evidence originating from research studies. Clinical epidemiologists in particular have developed criteria for appraising the published evidence regarding interventions available for clinical practice, the current standard probably being that produced by the Evidence-Based Medicine Working Group (Oxman et al., 1993; Guyatt et al., 1993, 1994). These guidelines are designed for the assessment of individual articles. They identify the dimensions to be considered and specify desirable attributes, but do not provide weights for individual dimensions or a formula for arriving at an overall evaluation of the article, much less the overall weight of evidence regarding an intervention. The guidelines are intended to assist the clinician in the management of individual patients and are concerned mainly with efficacy (performance under ideal conditions) and somewhat with effectiveness (performance under real-world conditions). Although the objective of placing clinical practice on a more scientific basis is entirely admirable, Maynard (1997) has argued that the evidence-based movement constitutes a return to the bad old days of the master clinician, who ignored efficiency and patient choice. The Critical Appraisal Skills Programme at Oxford has slightly adapted the clinical guidelines for use in health-care management and policy decisions (Muir Gray, 1997), although the focus is more on the former. The distinction between the needs of clinical practice and health care decision making is illustrated by the simultaneous appearance of two parallel publications from Oxford, one for each purpose (Sackett et al., 1997; Muir Gray, 1997). Box 5-1 presents the checklist offered for appraising randomized controlled trials (RCTs) for use in health care and policy decisions.

By and large, clinical epidemiologists take the position that only randomized studies are worth considering, a fairly reasonable position since randomized designs are usually feasible for interventions directed at individuals. Using nonrandomized designs in clinical evaluative research is therefore not generally defensible, although the health care criteria acknowledge the contribution of cohort studies and provide criteria for their evaluation (Muir Gray, 1997:91). *Outcomes research* represents another school of thought on determining the effects of clinical interventions, this one being based on observational data in administrative databases. The assumption is that sophisticated statistical analyses can adequately adjust for confounding variables and for differences in severity and case mix. The approach has been promoted by the U.S. Agency for Health Care Policy and Research, especially through its Patient Outcomes Research Teams (PORTs), but is much criticized by methodologists (Muir Gray, 1997:118–9).

Box 5-1. Checklist for appraising randomized controlled trials for use in evidence-based health care (Muir Gray, 1997:82–3)

Are the results of the trial valid?

- Did the trial address a clearly focused issue, in terms of
    population studied,
    intervention given, and
    outcomes considered?
- Was the assignment of patients to treatments concealed?
- Were all patients who entered the trial properly accounted for at its conclusion
    Was follow-up complete?
    Were patients analyzed in the groups to which they were randomized?
- Were patients, health workers, and study personnel "blind" to treatment?
- Were the groups similar at the start of the trial?
- Aside from the experimental intervention, were the groups treated equally?

What were the results?

- How large was the treatment effect?
- How precise was the estimate of the treatment effect?

How applicable were the research findings?

- How wide were the confidence intervals?
- What were the exclusion and inclusion criteria?
- How similar were the patients in the trial to the "local" patient group?
- Could the quality of service provided in the trial be reproduced "locally"?

Many of the interventions that might be considered for health policies cannot be evaluated using randomized controlled trials for ethical, political, and feasibility reasons. For a national educational or insurance program, the country is the appropriate unit of randomization, which is obviously not feasible. For community-level interventions, a *community intervention trial* (Symposium on Community Intervention Trials, 1995) may be conducted, in which the unit of allocation is the community, and the effective sample size is extremely small (often one or two communities per intervention). During preparation of the Canadian Community Health Practice Guidelines (Gyorkos et al., 1994) it was necessary to accept a broader range of research results, including those arising from observational and even descriptive studies. The proposed U.S. Community Preventive Services Guidelines will no doubt face similar issues. Thus, the best available evidence often comes in the form of weaker, even pre-experimental, designs. It is often difficult to identify a suitable comparison group. Before-and-after designs are therefore common, but their internal validity is severely threatened by problems such as history (the specific events occurring between the pretest and posttest in addition to the experimental variable) and regression to the mean (Campbell and Stanley, 1963). Sometimes the only available comparison is to a projection of what would have happened in the absence of the intervention. The clinical and health care criteria therefore need to be recalibrated, for application of criteria from the clinical sector rarely provides sufficient evidence to justify action, even though decisions still need to be taken.

Apart from research design issues, clinical and health care criteria refer to interventions that might be applied to individuals but not to population level interventions such as regulations, media campaigns, or public health services. Since assessing the impact on the individual patient is paramount in the health care setting, issues such as access and costs are not mentioned explicitly in the corresponding criteria, although they may be explicit in the last question on whether the quality of service could be reproduced locally. Clearly, several of the criteria will require modification to increase their policy relevance, and additional criteria will be needed (see Section 5.3).

Despite these limitations, clinical and health care criteria can serve as useful starting points for evaluating individual research reports, even if they are not entirely satisfactory for policy purposes in their current form.

5.2 Synthesizing Evidence: Systematic Reviews and Meta-analysis

The process of making evidence-based policy requires the summarizing of research results, which are often confusing and contradictory.

Systematic Reviews

Systematic reviews, also known as overviews or research synthesis, have emerged as a powerful tool for summarizing the evidence on a research question (Mosteller and Colditz, 1996). They are addressed in this chapter because they are used mainly to assess efficacy and effectiveness of health care interventions. The Cochrane Collaboration, named in honor of Archie Cochrane, the epidemiologist who provided the intellectual basis for evidence-based medicine (Cochrane, 1972), has led the way in developing methods and producing high-quality systematic reviews. The Collaboration has produced the Cochrane Library, which includes the

Cochrane Database of Systematic Reviews, the Cochrane Controlled Trials Register, and the Cochrane Review Methodology Database, all available in electronic form. A systematic review differs from an old-fashioned review article mainly in the selection of the articles to be examined and in the use of uniform criteria to evaluate them; this type of review is thus a much less subjective exercise. Framing the question is crucial to obtaining valid and useful results. Assembly of the evidence is the most important step and involves such challenges as finding reports that appear only in the non-peer-reviewed literature (theses, agency reports) and dealing with publication bias, such as the alleged tendency of authors to submit and journal editors to publish positive and not negative results. After reports have been selected, they are subjected to rigorous review, using criteria similar to those described in Section 5.1. A meta-analysis (see below) may or may not be included. The findings are synthesized into a narrative report. Again, two virtually identical sets of criteria are available for assessing overviews—those from the Evidence-Based Medicine Working Group (Oxman et al., 1994) for clinicians and those from Muir Gray (1997) for health care decision makers. The latter are presented in Box 5-2; again, they refer only peripherally to efficiency and access.

Box 5-2. Checklist for appraising review articles for use in evidence-based health care (Muir Gray, 1997:74–5)

Are the results of the review valid?

- Did the review address a focused issue?
- Did the authors look for the appropriate sort of papers?
- Were the important, relevant studies included?
- Did the review's authors do enough to assess the quality of the included studies?
- If the results of the review have been combined, was it reasonable to do so?

What are the results?

- What is the overall result of the review?
- How precise are the results?

Will the results help locally?

- Can the results be applied to the local population?
- Were all important outcomes considered?
- Are the benefits worth the harms and costs?

Meta-analysis

Meta-analysis is a narrower concept, defined as "[t]he process of using statistical methods to combine the results of different studies" (Last,
1995:105), although in practice the term is used more broadly, sometimes
synonymously with systematic reviews. It has been described as "possibly the most important policy-related research method that has developed in the past two decades" (Goodman, 1998:229), and books have
been published on the topic (Petitti, 1994). Meta-analysis can be regarded
as a form of descriptive study that is analogous to conducting a survey, or
actually a census, since meta-analysis generally tries to assemble all the
credible evidence bearing on a question, rather than relying on a sample.
The individual studies are sometimes scored according to quality, with
greater weight being assigned to those judged likely to yield the best-
quality evidence. Muir Gray (1997) suggests that the criteria for a meta-
analysis should be more stringent than for a (qualitative) review and accordingly adds some additional criteria for overviews that contain a
meta-analysis (Box 5-3).

The major justifications for meta-analysis are twofold: (1) improving
the precision of an estimate, by combining the sample sizes from many
studies; and (2) resolving inconsistencies. The first of these is much better
developed, but the second may be more important. If it is believed that
the results of all the individual studies are estimates of the same population value, then any differences are assumed to be due to chance and the
task is simply to summarize these results. This is the *fixed effects* model, of
which the best known example is probably the standard Mantel-Haenszel
statistic: when applied to meta-analysis, the individual studies are analogous to the strata in a stratified analysis. If it is believed that the observed
differences between studies reflect true differences in the underlying parameters, or heterogeneity, but that calculation of a summary result is justified, then a *random effects* model is appropriate; here the analogy is to
multilevel analysis (see Section 4.4), with each study being treated as a

---

**Box 5-3. Additional criteria for assessing a meta-analysis (Muir Gray,
1997:76)**

- Was the searching technique limited to an electronic search of
  MEDLINE? (Undesirable)
- Are the results of the trials all or mostly pointing in the same
  direction? (Desirable)
- Are the trials in the meta-analysis all small trials? (Very undesir-
  able).

group (subpopulation) with no assumption that the associations among variables are the same in all studies. Application of this model requires the estimation of more parameters and therefore leads to a less precise estimate. But perhaps the heterogeneity is precious: some authorities suggest that the main motivation for conducting meta-analysis should be explanation of differences rather than production of a single "best" estimate (Greenland, 1994). Much more flexible analysis is possible if the meta-analyst has access to the original data from the reports, allowing analysis of individual patient data or "pooled analysis" (Samet and Burke, 1998), rather than having to rely on whatever summary results were published. Sensitivity analysis has an important role in testing the robustness of a result to changes in various assumptions (e.g., inclusion or exclusion of certain studies). The concept of cumulative meta-analysis, analogous to sequential clinical trials, is emerging (Lau et al., 1995).

Applicability of meta-analysis to results of observational studies
Systematic reviews are equally relevant to observational and intervention studies, but the same is not necessarily true of meta-analysis. In a randomized intervention study, randomization can be depended on to eliminate confounding in the long run, and meta-analysis can help to get closer to that goal by combining the results of several studies. The larger sample size produces a more precise result. But how applicable is meta-analysis to nonrandomized evidence? This question applies to both observational studies of causation and the many evaluations of programs and polices in which randomization is not feasible. Nonrandomized studies are much more subject to confounding, which is not at all addressed by combining the results of several studies: if all the studies are subject to the same confounding, then the final result will be confounded, even if based on a huge combined sample size. The result may be precisely wrong. Shapiro (1994) recommended that the meta-analysis of published nonexperimental data be abandoned. Others recommend that meta-analysis be performed, emphasizing the explanation of the heterogeneity rather than the calculation of a summary estimate (Egger et al., 1998) or using a random effects model (Mosteller and Colditz, 1996).

5.3 Assessing Suitability for Policy

Clinicians are concerned primarily with the effect of an intervention on their patients, who are already in care. Health care managers are concerned with all the patients presenting to an institution. Policymakers must be concerned with the whole population and with inevitable resource limitations. This means that issues like efficiency and coverage must be considered, along with the practicality of implementation. The pertinent literature contains relatively few evaluations of policies that might be adopted, so policy developers must cadge together evidence from a variety of sources. Box 5-4 proposes criteria for assessing interventions for possible inclusion in health policy; these criteria are intended to apply to the entire body of evidence regarding an intervention, not to individual studies. In fact, the concept of effectiveness can be argued to encompass all of efficacy, generalizability, feasibility, and potential coverage, especially if the latter is interpreted as community effectiveness; the two remaining criteria would then be *Effectiveness and Efficiency*, the title of Archie Cochrane's (1972) famous book. But this simplification may be somewhat strained, and usage by various authorities differs enough to warrant keeping the criteria separate. Addressing these issues involves the usual differences in thinking and terminology between disciplines and eras.

Efficacy

Efficacy is a prerequisite for effectiveness and must be evaluated first. The quality of evidence on efficacy provided by a research study depends most fundamentally on the study design or architecture, which determines the potential of a study to yield valid results, although it does not guarantee that this potential is actually achieved.

Two quite separate traditions exist for categorizing and evaluating research designs for evaluating interventions, developed in clinical epidemiology and the social sciences, respectively. The work of the Canadian Task Force on the Periodic Health Examination (1994) and the US Preventive Services Task Force (1996) illustrates the epidemiologic approach with its emphasis on randomized designs. The Canadian Task Force (1994:xxxvii) criteria are as follows:

Box 5-4. Proposed criteria for determining whether an intervention should be included in a health policy

- *Efficacy:* Is the intervention known to work under optimal conditions?
- *Effectiveness:* Is the intervention known to work under normal conditions?
- *Applicability:* Is the intervention likely to be effective in the target population for the proposed policy?
- *Efficiency:* Could the money be spent more productively on other interventions?
- *Feasibility:* Can the intervention be implemented, given the sociopolitical context?
- *Potential coverage:* Can the intervention reach the whole target population?

  I. Evidence obtained from at least one properly randomized controlled trial

II-1. Evidence obtained from well-designed controlled trials without randomization

II-2. Evidence obtained from well-designed cohort or case-control analytic studies, preferably from more than one center or research group

II-3. Evidence obtained from comparisons between times or places with or without the intervention

 III. Opinions of respected authorities, based on clinical experience, descriptive studies, or reports of expert committees.

In general, type I evidence is considered good evidence to support the inclusion or exclusion of an intervention in the periodic health examination, type II evidence is considered fair evidence, and type III evidence is considered poor evidence, leaving the decision to be made on other grounds.

Some authorities now include meta-analysis in the list, at or near the very top, especially those meta-analyses involving analysis of individual data, although this is controversial. For example, Hadorn et al. (1996) propose the following list for use in development of clinical guidelines:

1. Supportive evidence from well-conducted RCTs that included 100 patients or more, such as multicenter trial or meta-analysis with quality ratings

2. Supportive evidence from well-conducted RCTs or meta-analysis with quality ratings, with fewer than 100 patients

3. Supportive evidence from well-conducted cohort studies, such as prospective or retrospective studies, or meta-analysis thereof

4. Supportive evidence from a well-conducted case–control study

5. Supportive evidence from poorly controlled or uncontrolled studies (e.g., significantly flawed RCTs, observational studies with high potential for bias, or case series or reports)

6. Conflicting evidence with weight of evidence supporting the recommendation

7. Expert opinion.

Other lists place meta-analyses alone at the top, whereas others would place it much lower. Similarly, some authorities would include analyses of administrative databases (outcome research) in the list, perhaps after case–control studies.

Campbell and Stanley's (1963) categorization of research designs and the associated threats to validity exemplifies the social science approach, and with its emphasis on quasi-experimental designs and external validity may have more to offer the policy epidemiologist. The basic argument is that pre-experimental designs cannot offer valid comparisons, whereas experimental (randomized) designs have the potential to offer valid comparisons but often suffer from low external validity and feasibility; the very features that are introduced to avoid bias and confounding often create an artificial situation, which limits generalizability. Quasi-experimental designs are nonrandomized designs that try to offer valid comparisons through the addition of extra comparison groups or measurements; some have no analogue in clinical or epidemiologic research. Table 5-1 lists the designs most applicable in health circles along with the terminology used there; several other designs seem less applicable to health and are rarely if ever used in this area. The feasibility columns in the table are somewhat speculative and the validity columns are a rough summarization of Campbell and Stanley's assessment of the extent to which the designs protect against sources of invalidity. Note that Campbell and Stanley use a rather narrow definition of external validity, which refers to the extent to which the conduct of the research can compromise generalizability (e.g., interaction between testing and intervention), but not to the underlying characteristics of the population.

Given its elegant resolution of the ethical objections to RCTs, the regression-discontinuity design deserves more attention than it receives in health services research (Trochim, 1990). Subjects are ranked from least to greatest severity of need according to a preprogram test, and the treatment is provided to the half with the greatest severity. All subjects are then assessed on an outcome measure, the postprogram test, which is not necessarily the same test, and the results for the treatment and comparison groups are regressed separately on the preprogram results. If the intervention has no effect, then the two regression lines should be more or less continuous, whereas if it has an effect, then there should be a discontinuity at the boundary between the two. As presented by Dunn (1981:343), the group of very similar individuals near the cutoff point is entered into a tie-breaking experiment.

Effectiveness

The effectiveness of the component parts of a policy in achieving their objectives is fundamental and deserves special elaboration. *Effectiveness* refers to the performance of an intervention in practice (the "real world"). But many research evaluations, including most RCTs (the elite evaluations), evaluate *efficacy*, the performance of the intervention under ideal conditions. The border between the two is fuzzy, so it is sometimes hard to determine just what a study has evaluated; the mega-trials advocated by Peto et al. (1995) seem to come closer to addressing effectiveness.

The measurement iterative loop (Tugwell et al., 1985; see Section 1.4) decomposes the "community effectiveness" of clinical interventions into five components:

Community effectiveness of intervention(s) = efficacy × diagnostic
accuracy × provider compliance × patient compliance × coverage

Assessment of effectiveness involves assessment of all five components;
the clinical epidemiology literature (e.g., Sackett et al., 1991) addresses
at least the first four. By specifying community effectiveness and in-

Table 5-1. Research Designs for Evaluation of Health Interventions

Design	Layout[a]	Feasibility	Internal Validity	External Validity
Pre-experimental designs				
One-shot case study	X O	High	Low	Moderate
One-group pretest– posttest	O X O	Moderate to high	Low	Low
Static-group comparison	X O / O	Moderate	Low	Moderate
True experimental designs				
Pretest–posttest control group (randomized trial with pretests)	R O X O / R O O	Low	High	Low
Posttest-only control group (randomized trial without pretests)	R X O / R O	Low	High	Moderate
Quasi-experimental designs				
Nonequivalent control group (cohort study)	O X O / O O	Moderate	Moderate	Low
Time series	O O X O O	Moderate to high	Moderate	Low
Multiple time series	O O X O O / O O O O	Moderate	High	Low
Multiple groups pretest–posttest	O X O / O X O / etc.	Moderate to high	Moderate to high	Low
Regression- discontinuity	C O X O / C O O	Moderate	Moderate to high	Moderate

[a]O, observation; X, intervention; R, random allocation; C, allocation at a cutoff; separating line, absence of random allocation.

Source: Table adapted from Campbell and Stanley (1963:8,40,56), with permission.

cluding coverage in the definition, the iterative loop approaches the impact of clinical interventions the population (see Section 6.3), although it does not consider adverse effects or effect on other conditions. Diagnostic accuracy and provider compliance are usually not applicable to population-level interventions, and patient compliance is often not applicable.

Ideally, the literature will contain the results of demonstration studies, in which the intervention was mounted in the field, under less artificial conditions than in a RCT. When the available evidence addresses only efficacy, some judgment must be exercised to assess the likely generalizability of the intervention. How artificial were the conditions under which the research was conducted? How expert were the professionals who provided the interventions? Would the intervention "work" if the intervention were provided by ordinary professionals under more ordinary conditions? Were the participants in the trial so highly selected as to make them unrepresentative of the (reference) population from which they were drawn? The issue here is the applicability of the research findings to the reference population under ordinary conditions.

Applicability

Usually this part of assessment is labeled "generalizability," but there appear to be three uses of that term: (1) external validity, as noted under efficacy; (2) representativeness of the research participants, as noted under effectiveness; and (3) applicability of research results to different populations. The third usage is relevant here, thus the term applicability will be used to avoid confusion. It is particularly relevant to policy epidemiology, which frequently involves applying data from one population to another, raising the following questions: Will the results of the published research apply in the population for which policy is being developed? Was the population in which the research was conducted sufficiently similar to the population for which policy is being developed to ensure a reasonable chance that the results can be replicated? Clinicians worry about comparability with respect to age, sex, education, or other characteristics that could influence the outcome. Policy epidemiologists should also consider the characteristics of the health care system and even the culture. A policy that works in one system may not work in another, e.g., preventive policies that work with salaried physicians may not work under fee-for-service payment.

Efficiency

Assessment of efficiency falls mainly within the ambit of the economist, but the epidemiologist makes an essential contribution in assessing health outcomes and brings a population health perspective. The essence of economic analysis is assessment of the marginal benefits and marginal costs of an intervention, compared to an alternative intervention. Four types of economic analysis are usually identified, all expressing costs in dollars but differing in the way that outcomes are quantified (Drummond et al., 1987):

1. *Cost-minimization analysis,* in which the outcomes are known or assumed to be identical and only the costs are compared. These conditions are rarely met, so the approach is rarely useful to the health-policymaker.
2. *Cost-effectiveness analysis,* in which the outcomes are expressed in "natural" units, e.g., life-years saved or cases of a disease prevented. Obviously the resulting cost-effectiveness ratios have meaning only when compared to similarly defined ratios for other interventions, i.e., the outcomes must have the same metric. Comparisons across different conditions are therefore generally impossible.
3. *Cost-benefit analysis,* in which all outcomes are converted to monetary equivalents. This has the advantage of enabling comparisons to be made across different types of programs, even those intended for different conditions, but the problems of converting the health outcomes into monetary terms are often insuperable (see Economic Burden of Ill Health in Section 4.1).
4. *Cost-utility analysis,* in which the outcomes are expressed as quality-adjusted life years (QALYs) gained or some similar measure. In principle, this also allows comparison of programs that have widely differing outcomes, but without the artificiality of converting outcomes into monetary equivalents; it is therefore potentially the most valuable to the policymaker. The challenge in cost-utility analysis is that conversion of the various health benefits to health utilities requires assignment of a numerical value to all relevant health states (see Composite Measures of Health in Section 2.2).

Other issues in economic analysis include which costs to include, what time period to consider, and what discount rate to apply to the value of future costs and benefits. Even more important is the perspective from which the analysis is performed; for policy purposes, this should almost always be that of society, perhaps occasionally that of government. *Sensitivity analysis* is widely used to assess the sensitivity of the results to the various assumptions made. An example of use of efficiency criteria appears in Box 5-5.

The Evidence-Based Medicine Group's guidelines on health care recommendations (Guyatt et al., 1995; summarized in Box 5-6) consider a broader range of factors that still focus on efficiency. This approach is directed toward policymakers rather than clinicians at the bedside, and reflects several methodological developments: availability of systematic reviews, clearer definition of clinical significance, and incorporation of the role of chance error. The data requirements for this approach are obviously severe, and it is likely to be difficult to apply in many cases.

Feasibility

It may be concluded that an intervention will confer substantial benefit on the health of the population and that the cost is reasonable relative to other interventions. Therefore, the intervention probably should be implemented. But whether the intervention actually can be implemented depends upon a number of other factors. Implementation may not be fea-

---

Box 5-5. When should a new technology be adopted?

Laupacis et al. (1992, 1993) formulated recommendations for adoption of a new technology on the basis of the marginal cost per QALY. As shown in Box Figure 5-5-1, they categorize the evidence for adoption of the new technology as

1. Compelling: the new technology is equally or more effective and less costly than the current technology.
2. Strong: the new technology is more effective and costs less than $20,000/QALY gained, or the new technology is less effective but saves more than $100,000/QALY lost through its adoption.
3. Moderate: the new technology is more effective and costs $20,000–$100,000/QALY gained, or the new technology is less effective and saves $20,000-$100,000/QALY lost.
4. Weak: the new technology is more effective but costs more than $100,000/QALY gained, or the new technology is less effective and saves less than $20,000/QALY lost.
5. Compelling evidence for rejection: the new technology is less or equally effective, but is more costly than the technology currently in use.

The $20,000 and $100,000 cutoffs were selected on the basis of programs currently funded, i.e., decisions that society had already made. The higher cutoff for replacing an established program with a cheaper one was intended to reflect the reluctance of society to drop established therapies in favor of less effective but cheaper ones. The algorithm is based entirely on cost-effectiveness, although the authors refer to the need to consider factors like feasibility and social values. The proposals were criticized on technical grounds—Gafni and Birch (1993) proposed healthy life expectancy as an alternative to QALYs—and it was argued that asymmetry in cutoff points would inevitably lead to increased total costs of health care (Naylor et al., 1993).

(continued)

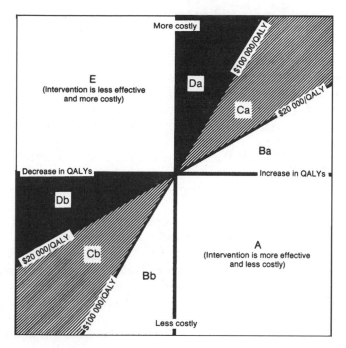

Box Figure 5-5-1. An algorithm for deciding when a new technology should be introduced. [Reprinted from How attractive does a new technology have to be to warrant adoption and utilization? Tentative guidelines for using clinical and economic evaluations by permission of the publisher, CMAJ, 1992; 146 (4), pp. 473–81.]

sible because the necessary resources such as expertise, equipment, or funding may be lacking. The intervention may not be compatible with the government's policy direction, which may be expressed in health goals. Or the intervention may simply be unacceptable to the public, in which case an educational program may be needed, as was the case with seat-belt legislation; to powerful interest groups, such as the commercial health insurance lobby in the United States; or to the politicians in power, who may reject harm reduction strategies proposed for problems such as illegal drug use. Published reports on the acceptability in similar jurisdictions may be available; if not, there may be a need to use expert opinion or public surveys.

Potential Coverage

This criterion refers to the extent that the intervention can reach its target population, if it is adapted as policy. Its dissemination could be limited by costs, distance, and communication difficulties, among others. For direct services programs potential coverage is related to access, and in general it is closely related to feasibility.

Box 5-6. A method for grading health care recommendations (Guy-att et al., 1995)

1. How strong is the evidence? Evaluation is based on:
   - Quality of evidence (RCT vs observational studies)
   - Presence or absence of important heterogeneity
2. How big an impact of treatment warrants its use? Evaluation is based on the threshold number needed to treat (TNNT), which is calculated from
   - Cost of treating the condition and the adverse effects of the therapy
   - Values (economic burden) of the target outcomes and adverse events
3. How much does the treatment work? The decision is based on
   - Relationship of observed NNT to threshold TNNT.

These few criteria incorporate a remarkable amount of information. To be considered important, heterogeneity must be both clinically important, with a difference of at least 20 percentage points between the point estimates of the two most disparate studies, or a gap of at least 5 percentage points between their confidence intervals, and it must be statistically significant ($P < 0.05$). The strength of the evidence is then graded as (1) RCT with no important heterogeneity; (2) RCT with important heterogeneity; and (3) Observational studies (with or without heterogeneity).

The number needed to treat (NNT; see Section 2.3) incorporates the absolute risk reduction. At the threshold NNT (TNNT), the total value of treatment inputs, which is the cost of treating TNNT patients and the resulting adverse effects (AE) less the cost of treating the one target event prevented, equals the total value of treatment outputs, or the value of having prevented one target event less the value of the adverse effects that the treatment caused. Mathematically,

$$(Cost_{treatment})(TNNT) + \Sigma\,[(Cost_{AE})(Rate_{AE})(TNNT)] - Cost_{target}$$
$$= Value_{target} - \Sigma\,[(Value_{AE})(Rate_{AE})(TNNT)]$$

from which it follows that:

$$TNNT = \frac{Cost_{target} + Value_{target}}{Cost_{treatment} + \Sigma\,\left[Rate_{AE}(Cost_{AE} + Value_{AE})\right]}$$

The final step assesses the magnitude of the intervention effect by comparing the confidence intervals of the observed NNT to the TNNT and leads to a judgment regarding the size of the effect:

continued

- Category 1 evidence: the confidence interval of the NNT does not overlap the TNNT. This is sufficient to make a definitive recommendation for or against adopting the intervention.
- Category 2 evidence: the confidence interval overlaps the TNNT. The recommendation (based on the point estimate) must be weaker.

Combining the ratings for strength of evidence and size of effect, the authors consider that A1 and B1 evidence to justify the strongest recommendations, A2 and B2, intermediate-strength recommendations, and C1 and C2, the weakest recommendations, showing the importance they attach to the research design.

Summary

Assessment of potential interventions begins with evaluation of individual studies and synthesis of the results of those studies. The commonly used criteria for assessment of individual studies relate mainly to clinical interventions; they focus on efficacy, which can usually be assessed by randomized controlled trials, and do not adequately address efficiency or other population-relevant criteria. Systematic reviews play an important role in summarizing the total body of evidence relating to an intervention, with meta-analysis providing a quantitative summary estimate of its effect. The applicability of meta-analysis to the observational evidence that is usually the best available for policy interventions may be limited. Suitability for policy should be determined on the basis of the entire body of available evidence. For population-level programs such as policies, randomized trial evidence is rarely available for assessment of efficacy; quasi-experimental evidence must then be the basis for policy decisions, and different criteria are needed. Assessment of effectiveness must consider whether the intervention can be applied by ordinary professionals to ordinary people, and is often more speculative. The epidemiologist collaborates with the economist in evaluating the efficiency of possible interventions, focusing on the effectiveness side of such analyses. It is necessary to consider the applicability of research results to the population for which the intervention is being considered. Equally important is the feasibility of implementing the intervention for the target population; here issues such as availability of necessary resources, conformity to national goals, and acceptability to the population come into play. Potential coverage considers whether the intervention can be applied to the whole population.

Key References

Guyatt GH, Sackett DL, Sinclair JC, et al., for the Evidence-Based Working Group. Users' Guides to the Medical Literature. IX. A method of grading health care recommendations. *JAMA* 1995;274:1800–4.

Mosteller F, Colditz GA. Understanding research synthesis (meta-analysis). *Annu Rev Public Health* 1996;17:1–23.

Muir Gray JA. *Evidence-based Healthcare: How to make health policy and management decisions.* New York: Churchill Livingstone, 1997.

6

Policy Choices

The health problems have been identified (Chap. 4) and the potential interventions assessed (Chap. 5)—now it is time to make decisions. At what level(s) should the disease be tackled: is prevention always to be preferred? Given that an intervention works, what will be its impact on the overall health of the population? With all the choices available to policymakers, how can they decide on priorities? Data can help inform these decisions, but eventually judgement must be exercised in making a final decision. This chapter continues the transformation of health information into health intelligence, the basis for decision making. The actual decisions will rarely be made by epidemiologists alone.

6.1 Prevention and Disease Control

Disease control can be attempted at several levels: prevention, cure, rehabilitation, or palliation. Epidemiology can help to select the optimal combination of approaches. Prevention warrants special attention, because societies say that they prefer to intervene as early in the course of a disease as possible, although their allocation of resources suggests that they are not quite convinced about this, and because epidemiologists claim to have special knowledge of it. Several levels of prevention are usually defined, although their boundaries are somewhat indistinct. Before we discuss prevention, however, we must address health promotion.

Health Promotion

Health promotion used to mean risk factor modification through health education, but now has a much broader meaning in most countries. The international health promotion movement grew out of the Health for All declaration of the World Health Organization (WHO) (1981a:11): "[T]he main social target of governments and of WHO should be the attainment by all the peoples of the world by the year 2000 of a level of health that will permit them to lead a socially and economically productive life." It soon became clear that this ambitious goal could be achieved only through a focus on the determinants of health. The European Region of

WHO saw health promotion as the route to health for all in developed countries. Its newly developed Office of Health Promotion (World Health Organization, 1986) defined health promotion as "the process of enabling people to increase control over, and to improve, their health. . . . [H]ealth promotion is not just the responsibility of the health sector, but goes beyond healthy life-styles to well-being." Accordingly, health promotion focuses on fostering positive health, as distinct from preventing disease, and on the broadest determinants of health. During the 1980s, health promotion became a major influence on public health and health policy in many countries. Its major statement has been the 1986 Ottawa Charter on Health Promotion (World Health Organization, 1986), which identified five approaches for health promotion: (1) develop personal skills; (2) strengthen community action; (3) create supportive environments; (4) reorient health services; and (5) build healthy public policy.

These are to be accomplished through the processes of enabling, mediation, and advocacy. The movement has been led primarily by social scientists, and epidemiology may contribute especially to the difficult problems of measurement and evaluation.

Primordial Prevention

The term primary prevention is usually used to refer to attempts at preventing a disease from ever occurring, i.e., to reduce the incidence of the disease. This would seem to include health promotion (although health promoters include preventive and other health services within health promotion). Terminology is elastic: should the term be confined to interventions directed at specific diseases (e.g., immunization), or should it also include general approaches? Several decades ago, Leavell and Clark (1965:20) distinguished between two types of primary prevention: (general) health promotion and protection against specific diseases. More recently, Rose (1985) distinguished between the determinants of cases of disease in individuals and the determinants of the levels or incidence of diseases in populations, pointing out that there are widely different distributions of certain risk-factors in different populations, e.g., virtually the entire Finnish population had high-risk cholesterol levels, by Asian standards. Perhaps building on Rose's distinctions, Beaglehole et al. (1993:86) define *primordial prevention* as avoiding "the emergence and establishment of the social, economic and cultural patterns of living that are known to contribute to an elevated risk of disease"; they appear to reserve "primary prevention" for interventions directed at specific diseases. The *Dictionary of Epidemiology* (Last 1995:131) offers a slightly different perspective on primordial prevention: "This term is advocated by some authors to describe elimination of risk factors, precursors, genetic counselling to avoid genetically determined conditions, etc., in contrast to primary prevention by reducing risks of exposure." Although boundaries will always be fuzzy, definition of primordial prevention as a separate level of prevention seems a useful clarification. Primordial prevention overlaps with health promotion and has great relevance to the emerging field of population health (see Section 1.5). Like these fields, it will be very difficult to implement and evaluate. Currently the evidence for its effectiveness is based mainly on studies of inequalities in health and its determinants among population groups. Epidemiologists can contribute to determining the effectiveness of primordial prevention by conducting such studies and by including environmental and other "fundamental" determinants of health in their etiological research.

Primary Prevention

Beaglehole et al. (1993:88) define *primary prevention* as limiting the incidence of disease by controlling causes and risk factors, whereas the *Dictionary* (Last, 1995:130) offers a more general definition: "[T]he protection of health by personal and communitywide effects, e.g., preserving good nutritional status, physical fitness, and emotional well-being, immunizing against infectious diseases, and making the environment safe." The archetypal examples of primary prevention are immunization and environmental hygiene (pasteurization of milk, chlorination of water). For chronic disease, primary prevention usually amounts to risk factor modification. It is available only when at least some risk factors are known, although detailed knowledge of etiology is not always necessary. There are two classic approaches.

The *high-risk strategy* identifies the individuals in a population who are at high-risk for disease and concentrates on modifying their risk factors. It targets those individuals who will benefit most from such modifications, thus having the potential to be especially cost-effective, avoids bothering those who will benefit least, and fits well with patterns of medical practice. Usually it targets those individuals with the highest levels of exposure to, e.g., smoking and indolence, but in the case of alcohol consumption, where risk is minimal at moderate consumption levels, it could be argued that both extremes of consumption should be targeted. The approach necessitates identifying high-risk individuals, as exemplified by the United States approach to cholesterol lowering, with its call for everyone to "know your number." This means testing the entire population, with attendant costs, worries, and false positives. It labels people who test positive as abnormal, then asks them to behave abnormally for their social environment, e.g., to eat differently from their peers. More important, the distribution of most risk factors is not bimodal but unimodal, so the distinction between risk categories is not clear. It usually turns out that most cases of disease occur in low- or moderate-risk people, who are by far the most numerous but who gain no benefit from the high-risk approach (see the hypothetical example in Box 6-1). If used alone, the approach is therefore doomed to have little effect in most cases.

The *population strategy* targets the entire population, attempting to

---

Box 6-1. Most cases occur in low-risk people

The exposed group in Box 2.3 actually had three levels of exposure:

Exposure Level	Prevalence	Incidence	RR	pRR	Proportion of all Disease
Nil	0.60	0.030/year	1.00	0.60	0.43 ⎫
Low	0.25	0.048/year	1.60	0.40	0.29 ⎬ 0.72
Intermediate	0.10	0.060/year	2.00	0.20	0.14
High	0.05	0.120/year	4.00	0.20	0.14
TOTAL	1.00	(0.042/year)	(1.40)	1.40	1.00

The population attributable fraction = $(1.40 - 1.00)/1.40 = 0.29$, as before. This is not surprising, since the RR of 2.0 in Box 2–3 is the weighted average of the RRs in this box.

The last column (above) indicates the proportion of all disease that occurs at each level of exposure. Note that 72% of all cases of the disease occur among people with zero or low levels of "exposure"; these cases would have been missed by a preventive program using the high-risk approach.

---

move the population distribution in the direction of lower risk. Rose made the case for this approach in a famous paper (1985) and a book (1992), noting that a large number of people exposed to a low risk may generate more cases than a small number of people exposed to a high risk. He argued that a population strategy is necessary whenever risk is widely diffused though the whole population: "[M]ass diseases and mass exposures require mass remedies" (Rose 1992:95). He pointed out that the approach is radical—it gets to the root of the problem—powerful, since it reduces everyone's risk; and appropriate, inasmuch as it does not label anyone as abnormal. It also causes the prevalence of high-risk individuals in the population to fall, since "the visible part of the iceberg (prevalence) is a function of its total mass (the population average)" (Rose 1992:72). A disadvantage is that even low-risk people are urged to change their health behaviors. People with cholesterol values that are low by North American standards may yet benefit, but they will only benefit a little, and thus the approach encounters the *prevention paradox*: that "a preventive measure that brings large benefits to the community offers little to each participating individual" (Rose 1992:12). The approach is exemplified by the Ontario report on cholesterol, which on the basis of the evidence then available rejected the idea of testing the whole population (Toronto Working Group on Cholesterol Policy, 1989).

As with most sharp dichotomies, neither approach has a monopoly on truth. The approaches are often complementary, in that people at very high risk may need to be identified to benefit from intensive intervention, even when a (less intensive) population strategy has been adopted. Epidemiology can help to find the appropriate balance by projecting the results of each approach on to the population and perhaps by formal disease modeling.

Secondary Prevention

Secondary prevention comprises early detection and intervention, in the belief that this will yield better results than waiting for a disease to present in its usual fashion. Thus, the objective is not to reduce incidence but to prevent the development of full-blown disease and thereby reduce the case fatality from the disease (Morrison, 1992). The time between the detection of the case by an early-detection program and the point at which it would present in the absence of such a program is the *lead time*.

Again there are terminological problems: cardiologists refer to secondary prevention of myocardial infarction as attempts to prevent a second myocardial infarction in patients who have already had a first infarction, whereas most epidemiologists would call this tertiary prevention (both parties would agree that attempts to prevent the first infarction constitute primary prevention). Leavell and Clark (1965: 20) acknowledged both uses when they broke down secondary prevention into early diagnosis/prompt treatment and disability limitation. The distinctions among levels of prevention can be blurred in other ways: one could argue that early detection and intervention to modify a risk factor, which most people would call secondary prevention, constitutes primary prevention of the actual disease, using the high-risk approach. When early detection is attempted in a free-standing population without symptoms of the disease in question it is referred to as *screening*: "Screening for disease control can be defined as the examination of asymptomatic people in order to classify them as likely, or unlikely, to have the disease that is the object of the screening" (Morrison 1992:3). Screening programs may fail to follow up persons who test positive, and for this reason *case-finding* is sometimes advised. Here the early detection is attempted among persons who are visiting a health professional for another reason, as when a physician decides to check the blood pressure of every patient who visits her, regardless of the reason for the visit. The advantage is the built-in follow-up. Muir Gray (1997:47) presents another definition of case-finding: testing of asymptomatic persons who are at risk through being related to a person with a disease.

False positives are the Achilles's heel of screening programs: since the vast majority of individuals tested do not have the target disease, even a highly specific test will produce many more false positives than true positives, and thus a low positive predictive value. For this reason, screening is often conducted among high-risk groups, in whom the prevalence of the disease is higher.

Early detection is subject to at least two major biases that can make it appear more effective than it really is: *length bias,* the tendency to identify indolent cases that would usually continue to progress slowly in the absence of intervention, and *lead time bias,* which confuses the early diagnosis (lead time) with increased survival. Obviously a screening program can be successful only if it can detect early cases, which is much harder than detecting full-blown clinical cases, and if these cases are provided with interventions that are effective in improving the outcome; similarly, screening for risk factors should be confined to *reversible* risks (Rose 1992:38).

The only really satisfactory approach to evaluating a screening program for a fatal disease is a randomized controlled trial with death as the outcome. Since few such trials have been conducted of screening programs, criteria (summarized in Box 6-2) have been developed for determining when early detection is indicated. For the policymaker, the question is whether to introduce a population screening program (Wilson and Jungner, 1968). As presented for clinicians by Sackett et al. (1991:153–70), the question is when the clinician should seek an earlier diagnosis. Remarkably few diseases meet the criteria for screening for early disease, cancer of the breast and cervix, hypertension, and certain conditions of the newborn being the best examples.

Epidemiology can help to assess the case for secondary prevention by calculating predictive values and modeling the effects of the program on the health of the population.

Box 6-2. Criteria for screening programs (adapted from various sources)

- Disease
  Imposes significant burden (frequency, severity)
  Significant detectable preclinical period (DPCP)
  Earlier treatment offers improved prognosis
- Test
  Valid (adequate sensitivity and specificity)
  Cheap
  Safe
  Acceptable to population
- Health care system
  Test reaches those at substantial risk
  Follow-up of positive tests provided
  Resources sufficient to provide intervention to the newly discovered cases

Tertiary Prevention

This term usually refers to the prevention of disability or complications in persons who already have established disease. It thus includes good-quality medical care and rehabilitation as well as the clinical definition of secondary prevention; Leavell and Clark (1965:20) equated it to rehabilitation. The resulting labeling of virtually all curative and rehabilitative care as prevention seems unhelpful, so tertiary prevention will not be further treated here.

Cost-effectiveness of Prevention

Proponents once offered prevention as the answer to rising health care costs, and politicians still make that claim on occasion. But a number of critics, led by Russell (1986), have questioned this claim. Bonneux et al. (1998) show that by preventing early deaths prevention may allow more people to reach old age with its higher prevalence of disease and thus may actually *increase* health care costs in the long run (see also the example of cancer in Box 2-2). The same is true for eliminating cigarette smoking (Barendregt et al., 1997). A consensus seems to be emerging that prevention should be practiced to reduce the occurrence of disease and death, not to save money. As Rose (1992:4) puts it, "[i]t is better to be healthy than ill or dead. That is the beginning and the end of the only real argument for preventive medicine. It is sufficient."

When to Prevent?

In principle, the earlier the intervention the better, in that it will then prevent the most morbidity and mortality, but things will not necessarily work out this way in practice. The policymaker must consider the costs of prevention at each level, and also the failures, since these will require re-intervention at later stages. Disease modeling (Gunning-Schepers, 1989) may help to weigh the costs and benefits of the various approaches and to target efforts.

Gunning-Schepers (1995) suggests that the decision to mount a prevention program should be based on the following factors:

1. The importance for public health of avoiding the problem, or the frequency and severity of the problem
2. The importance for public health of the intervention, or its probable impact
3. The importance for public health of avoiding a more expensive intervention; this is related to the cost-effectiveness of the intervention
4. The importance for public health of maintaining the preventive effort, (including support of other preventive efforts)
5. Pressure from politicians, the population, and the health care system.

6.2 Predicting the Effect of a Policy on a Population

Decisions regarding health policy must take into consideration a large number of variables concerning populations, determinants of health, diseases, and interventions. Disease modeling can help to assess the influence of all these variables and to predict what would happen as a result of (combinations of) interventions. It can be undertaken at various levels of complexity.

Predicting Health Trends in the Absence of Intervention

A first step is determining the trend of events in the absence of any (new) intervention. Three approaches are possible:

Statistical

This approach does not attempt to separate the influences of demographic and risk factors, although both may be implicit in the projections. Past trends are extrapolated into the future, using methods ranging from simple linear extrapolation through various transformations and statistical distributions to sophisticated models encompassing cyclical patterns, e.g., ARIMA (Helfenstein, 1991). Flanders (1995) reports that the binomial, Poisson, and exponential distributions often yield similar results when modeling disease occurrence. Unfortunately, the choice among models is not always made on entirely rational grounds (see Box 6-3). As a rule, extrapolation should only be carried out for up to the period of time for which past data are available (Ruwaard et al., 1994:120).

Demographic

The aging of the population has major implications for its health status, given the relation between age and health. Demographic models are extremely important at the policy level, because public policy deals with

---

Box 6-3. The contribution of Goldilocks to statistical modelling

In the early days of HIV/AIDS, an important committee tried to estimate the future incidence of AIDS, working from about 5 years of data. First they tried the logistic model, but the result was "too low" to be credible; naturally it suggested that the growth rate had stopped increasing and that the incidence would shortly level off. Then they tried the exponential model, which predicted rapid and increasing incidence. This result was "too high," and was unacceptable to politicians because it would frighten the public. Then they tried the polynomial model, which yielded an intermediate result and was concluded to be "ju-u-ust right"!

Box 6-4. Demographic modeling of health care

In the 1980s, the Canadian Medical Association's Task Force on the Allocation of Health Care Resources (1984) projected then current rates of institutional care onto the future Canadian population and predicted alarmingly high utilization, requiring, for example, the construction of almost 1000 new chronic care hospitals by the year 2021, more than doubling the then existing supply. The report was roundly criticized for artificiality by some academics, but it captured the attention of the government and the media! It was also very useful in demonstrating that something had to be changed in patterns of elder care.

---

populations. Furthermore, much is known about demographic trends: most of the people who will be affected by disease in the next few decades have already been born, and it is negligent not to use this information. This approach starts from population projections (Section 3.3), to provide a picture of the future age and sex composition of the population. Current age- and sex-specific rates of the disease are applied to these future populations, assuming that these rates remain unchanged. Such projections are useful in isolating the effects of demographic change, but because they ignore all other factors they are unlikely to prove correct. Box 6-4 provides an example of the demographic approach.

Epidemiologic
This approach considers changes in the prevalence of risk factors. It requires knowledge of those risk factors, the associated relative risks (RRs), recent and future trends in their prevalence, and the causal model—the way in which two or more risk factors work together to cause a disease, specifically whether their effects are additive, multiplicative, or otherwise. Unfortunately, this information is rarely known, and it is common for models to make simplifying assumptions, usually that a multiplicative model applies and that the risk factors are distributed independently in the population. The calculations turn out to involve the formula for the impact fraction (IF; see Section 2.3):

$$\text{IF} = \frac{I_1 - I_2}{I_1} = 1 - \frac{I_2}{I_1} = 1 - \frac{\Sigma p_2 \text{RR.} I_\text{U}}{\Sigma p_1 \text{RR.} I_\text{U}} = 1 - \frac{\Sigma p_2 \text{RR}}{\Sigma p_1 \text{RR}}$$

where subscripts 1 and 2 refer to the situations before and after a change in the prevalence of the risk factors, and the summation is across the levels of exposure. Solving the first version of the formula for I_2 and then inserting the last version for IF we arrive at

$$I_2 = I_1 (1 - IF) = I_1 \left(\frac{\Sigma p_2 RR}{\Sigma p_1 RR} \right)$$

Box 6-5 provides an example of epidemiologic modeling, based on the earlier example of Box 6-1. Models using the impact fraction or its variants, the population attributable fraction and the population preventive fraction, are inherently static in that they fail to recognize the changes that occur in the underlying population.

Combinations

Various combinations of these approaches are possible and take us into the realm of disease modeling (see below). There is potential for double-counting of effects when statistical extrapolations of disease trends, which presumably reflect trends in risk factors, are combined with epidemiologic projections, which are explicitly based on changes in risk factors.

Box 6-5. Impact of reducing exposure to a risk factor

An intervention program in the population described in Box 6-1 has now reduced exposure levels to those in column p_2. What is the expected effect on the incidence of the disease?

Exposure Level	Prevalence Before (p_1)	Incidence Before (I_1)	RR	p_1RR	Prevalence After (p_2)	p_2RR
Nil	0.60	0.030/year	1.00	0.60	0.85	0.85
Low	0.25	0.048/year	1.60	0.40	0.10	0.16
Intermediate	0.10	0.060/year	2.00	0.20	0.04	0.08
High	0.05	0.120/year	4.00	0.20	0.01	0.04
TOTAL	1.00	(0.042/year)	1.40	1.40	1.00	1.13

$$\text{Impact Fraction (IF)} = 1 - \frac{\Sigma p_2 RR}{\Sigma p_1 RR} = 1 - \frac{1.13}{1.40} = 0.193 = 19.3\%$$

$$I_2 = I_1(1 - IF) = 0.042(1 - 0.193) = 0.034$$

If the exposure causes the disease, then the incidence will eventually be reduced by 19.3%; incidence after the intervention will be 80.7% of that before the intervention, or 0.034 cases/person-year.

The Public Health Status and Forecasts report (Ruwaard et al., 1994:99 ff.) made several types of projections of future health status, described as

- demographic, acknowledging that population projections already make certain assumptions regarding future trends in overall mortality;
- epidemiologic, our "statistical" approach, using ARIMA models to extrapolate past trends in disease-specific morbidity and mortality and superimposing them on demographic trends;
- exploratory, our "epidemiologic" approach, encompassing changes in exposures to risk factors.

Similar projections were made for health care utilization.

Expansion versus compression of morbidity

Major disagreement exists regarding future trends in morbidity: will there be contraction as the population's health improves or expansion as the population ages? The debate began with a classic paper by Fries (1980), who noted that the survival curve is becoming rectangular as an increasing proportion of the population reaches the biological life span of about 85 years, and argued that most of the extra life years could be lived in good health: prevention could compress any apparently inevitable period of illness into an increasingly shorter period of time. This generally optimistic scenario has been rebutted by other studies (Bonneux et al., 1998). The Public Health Status and Forecasts report examined recent Dutch trends in healthy life expectancy (Ruwaard et al., 1994:62, 118) and found compression of morbidity in middle-aged males but no trend in other age–sex groups. It projected a tendency toward expansion of morbidity in the future. For the effect of eliminating a cause of death, see the example in Box 2-2.

Health and Disease Modeling

Definition

Disease modeling refers to attempts to express patterns of disease occurrence in the form of mathematical relationships so that they may be summarized or projected into the future. The term encompasses a wide range of activities, from simple to very complex, but is used here to refer to programs that incorporate at least changes in populations and risk factor prevalence. Initially developed for modeling epidemics of communicable disease, it is now being applied to chronic disease and even to health. Sophisticated modeling has only become feasible with the availability of substantial computing power and is more highly developed in economics and engineering than in health. Its terminology has not yet become stable; indeed, it is still uncertain what activities should be included within the heading.

Uses

Disease modeling provides a way of projecting research results onto a population, integrating a whole range of data into a scenario. The exercise may be carried out for various purposes:

- Description or explanation, to help interpret events, understand relationships, and identify disadvantaged groups
- Prediction, to predict future patterns and the effects of potential interventions
- Technology assessment, to predict the impact of a new technology in situations where direct evaluation is impractical
- Support for decision making, through answering "what if?" questions, such as the following: If the prevalence of smoking were reduced by 30%, what would be the impact on mortality or on Alzheimer's disease (for which smoking may be protective)? If lowering cholesterol increases cancer or trauma rates while reducing cardiovascular risks, what would be its overall impact on the population's health? Disease modeling is particularly useful for comparing the projected impact of alternative scenarios and for finding the optimal combination of interventions.
- Communication of complex issues, through use of graphics and examples
- Teaching of epidemiologic concepts
- Development of new knowledge, by combining facts and insights from a variety of sources.

Advantages

Development of a model encourages precise language and orderly thinking, forces quantification, imposes consistency on data from different times and different places, exposes assumptions, enables one to test which assumptions are critical, and helps to detect gaps in knowledge. Most important, disease modeling can deal with more variables than the human mind can consider at a single time, e.g., models can deal simultaneously with multifactorial interventions and the effect of varying age structures of population. This allows models to reflect the dynamic nature of changes in health. Some even incorporate the role of chance.

Limitations

All disease modelers bemoan the lack of adequate data, especially those regarding the causal model and the joint distribution of risk factors. The result is that models must incorporate a great many assumptions, the implications of which may be hard to assess. Some models are too ambitious, trying to model every possible variable. It is generally better to attempt a minimally predictive model that contains only key variables and processes, and acknowledge that no single model, however complicated, can answer all questions.

Types of models
Several useful distinctions can be made, although few are black and white.

Statistical epidemiologic models and mathematical biological models. Epidemiologic models show the occurrence of disease in a population and are most relevant to health policy. Biological models show the underlying processes in individuals (e.g., multistage models of carcinogenesis), and are most relevant to understanding disease causation.

Deterministic and stochastic models. Deterministic models use formulas to calculate a single estimate, with or without confidence intervals; given the same input data they produce the same result every time they are used. Stochastic models use probabilities to simulate the experience of a large number of individuals and produce a different distribution of results each time they are used; their incorporation of chance variation makes the results more realistic and thus occasionally bizarre.

Macro- and microsimulation models. The contrast between these two models seems the most fundamental distinction, from a methodological point of view. Macrosimulation, or cell-based, models are similar to traditional epidemiologic approaches and thus have the advantage of using familiar concepts like relative risks and attributable fractions. They model phenomena at the population level by dividing the population into categories representing all possible combinations of time, demographic characteristics, and risk factors, applying the appropriate relative risks and rates to each category, and then aggregating the results for individuals across the entire population. They are usually deterministic, but can also be stochastic. Such models are prone to assorted biases, mainly because of their inherent assumptions, and are cursed by multidimensionality (too many cells to deal with). Microsimulation (state-event, Markov) models begin with a hypothetical cohort of individuals, often newborns, and proceed to simulate the life trajectory of each individual on the basis of conditional probabilities of moving from one state to another. A cross-sectional look can be taken across the population at any age or year, to assess health status. Although usually stochastic, microsimulation models can also be deterministic. Microsimulation does not assume a causal model, but it does require a huge numbers of conditional probabilities. A microsimulation model is a completely disaggregated macrosimulation model, so any microsimulation can be rewritten as a macrosimulation, but the reverse is not true.

Disease-specific and comprehensive modeling. Enough is known to support modeling of only a few diseases: cardiovascular disease, a few cancers, and a very few injuries. Modeling the overall health of a population must therefore confine itself to selected diseases, lumping "all other" diseases into a residual category. It must also consider competing risks, the effect of changes in mortality from one disease on the occurrence of other diseases (see Section 2.1). For well-studied risk factors such as smoking, it may be possible to ignore specific diseases and model overall mortality, but this loses a great deal of detail.

Mortality and morbidity. Mortality is easier to model because it involves a single stage and a wealth of mortality data is available. But relative risks may be harder to find for mortality than for incidence, and the model results will be subject to the same limitations as the mortality data on which they are based (see Section 3.4). Morbidity models must estimate prevalence as well as incidence, and this introduces tremendous complexity, i.e., the need to incorporate survival experience and both risk and prognostic factors. Furthermore, there are important limitations in the availability of incidence, prevalence and survival data.

Clinical and policy models. Clinical models are designed to provide guidance for clinical decision making, whereas policy or public health models attempt to provide guidance for policymakers. The former seek to reproduce the health of an individual suffering from heart disease, renal failure, etc. and predict the effects of a treatment regimen for research or educational purposes. Policy models must have a population health perspective, recognizing changes in the composition of the population and considering the dispersion and cost-effectiveness of interventions. It is important for these models to consider the overall health status of the population, e.g., all-causes mortality, rather than modeling a single cause. If they are to be used as intended, such models must be timely and relevant to government priorities.

Processes. Processes to be modeled may include disease occurrence, primary prevention, secondary prevention, treatment, and overall disease control.

Box 6-6 provides several examples of disease models.

Validation of models

Validation is essential, but presents problems similar to those of validating tests or research instruments: if we knew the truth, we would not need the model. Model validation should be separated from model development, and should use different data. A model should be good enough to serve its purpose, but need not be perfect.

6.3 Priority Setting

Policymakers need to determine what topics to address, and in what order. Like the rest of policymaking, priority setting is part science and

Box 6-6. Examples of disease models

Prevent (Gunning-Schepers, 1989) is a cell-based, macrosimulation public health model of the impact of changes in the prevalence of risk factors on mortality rates. In its original form, it modeled eight diseases: lung cancer, chronic obstructive lung disease, ischemic heart disease: cerebrovascular accidents, cirrhosis, accidental falls, motor vehicle crashes, and breast cancer on the basis of five risk factors: smoking, hypertension, cholesterol, alcohol, and obesity. Herbert (1994) developed an Ontario database for the model and added seatbelt use as an additional risk factor. Input data are required for

- population, including size, birth rates, and past trends therein;
- mortality rates from all causes and from the specific causes modeled;
- risk factors, including prevalence and trends, relative risk for each risk factor-disease combination; lag time between cessation of exposure and achievement of maximum reduction in risk; and latent time between a change in incidence and a change in mortality.

On the basis of this information, the program projects "autonomous trends" in mortality for up to 50 years from established trends in risk factors in the absence of intervention. The user is then invited to specify certain "interventions," which are actually changes in risk factor prevalence that can be expected as the result of interventions, and the program calculates a new set of projections, incorporating the interventions as well as the autonomous trends. A wide range of outputs is available, including survival curves, life expectancy, and general and cause-specific mortality.

The *Harvard cardiovascular policy model* (Weinstein et al., 1987) models a single disease category but incorporates morbidity and treatment. It has three components: a demographic/epidemiologic model forecasts incidence, a bridge model estimates short-term outcomes, and a disease history model estimates long-term outcomes. The model has been used to explain the observed reductions in mortality from coronary heart disease (Hunink et al., 1997).

Can-Trol (Eddy, 1986) projects the incidence of various cancers according to population and risk factor trends. It was used to set targets for the U.S. Healthy People initiative.

The *Harvard incidence–prevalence model* was used in the World Bank's Global Burden of Disease project to describe relations among incidence, recovery, mortality, and fatality. Murray and Lopez (1994) point out that because of the interdependence of these variables, one can start from the most secure data and estimate the others.

POHEM (POpulation health expectancy model; Wolfson, 1994) is a public health microsimulation model developed at Statistics Canada. In

continued

place of relative risks and risk factor prevalences, POHEM requires a large set of transitional probabilities indicating the probability that an individual will move from one condition to another (single to married, non-smoking to smoking, healthy to diseased, etc.) at each time. It draws upon the Harvard cardiovascular policy model and the Framingham logistic equation. Starting from a hypothetical birth cohort, the program develops a branching structure to generate the life histories of these individuals.

A global microsimulation model has been developed at Erasmus University (Bonneux et al., 1995) and adapted to several specific diseases and uses.

MISCAN (Oortmarssen et al., 1990) is also a microsimulation model, developed specifically to evaluate breast and cervical cancer screening programs, and later expanded to prostate and colorectal cancer.

The *resource allocation framework* (Angus et al., 1995) is an attempt to model the entire Canadian health care system; it will be described in Section 7.2, Resource Allocation.

---

part politics; epidemiology can contribute to the science, which can be undertaken at several different degrees of sophistication. But priorities will also be influenced by the agency mission, political climate, feasibility, and other factors. The evidence base for evaluating the options is often weak, and it is up to the epidemiologist to assess that knowledge and to make the best possible recommendations. This section addresses three issues: the contribution of health data, the contribution of public input, and the group process necessary to arrive at a final decision.

Uses of Health Data in Priority Setting

Prioritizing diseases or other health problems

We begin with the relatively simple problem of prioritizing diseases solely on the basis of frequency or disease burden (of course, other aspects may be equally important, and will be addressed later). Choosing among health problems is relatively easy if all the data are of one type (e.g., numbers of deaths), since the candidates can simply be ranked. The situation is more difficult when the outcomes cut across several dimensions, e.g., deaths, hospital days, and disability. The Dutch Public Health Status and Forecasts project (Ruwaard et al., 1994:53 ff.) simply prepared separate lists of the top 10 diseases with respect to potential years of life lost (PYLL), prevalence (mainly chronic diseases), and incidence (mainly acute diseases); after eliminating duplications this yielded a total of 25 priority diseases and disorders. Measures such as quality-adjusted life years (QALY) and disability-free life expectancy (Section 2.2) offer a better solution by integrating several factors, as might estimates of the economic burden of ill health (Section 4.1).

Prioritizing risk factors

When programs are directed against risk factors the situation is more complex, since risk factors are important only because of their effects on health outcomes. The population attributable fraction (PAF) can be used to estimate the proportion of a health problem that is attributable to a specific risk factor (see Section 2.3 and Box 6-7).

The two approaches in Box 6-7 can be combined to estimate the total number of deaths (or other health events) from all causes that can be attributed to each risk factor (attributable mortality or morbidity [AM]), as shown in Table 6-1. This information shows which risk factor modification program would have the biggest impact on the health of the population and could serve as the effectiveness side of a cost-effectiveness analysis of alternative programs. Table 6-1 is directly applicable only in the artificial case in which risk factors can be eliminated; a more realistic approach would use the impact fraction to reflect their reduction. The methodological problems are great, especially in accounting for the effects of confounding and effect modification when there is multifactorial causation. Other questions to be considered include the following: How hard will it be to achieve the risk factor modification? Can the theoretical improvements be achieved? Removal of a risk factor may not lower risk to that of the never-exposed. Will the prevented deaths simply be replaced by deaths from other causes—the issue of competing risks? What will it cost to prevent the deaths? The situation is much more satisfactory when a validated disease model is available, e.g., Prevent (see Section 6.2).

Prioritizing interventions

The key criterion for prioritizing interventions should usually be their impact when included in a policy, i.e., their effect on the health of a whole population. *Health impact assessment* has been defined as "any combination of procedures or methods by which a proposed policy or program may be judged as to the effect(s) it may have on the health of a population" (Frankish et al., 1996:7). Thus, health impact assessment is about predicting the impact of a policy before its introduction, as distinct from evaluating its impact after implementation (Section 8.1). Health impact assessment aims to achieve health gain: "the result of a systematic process of approving, for a specific population, a range of measures that are based on the length of life and quality of life, and then providing and planning health resources that increase the average length of improved life enjoyed by that population" (World Health Organization, 1994). Will the population accept the policy, or adhere to (comply with) the program? How big an effect is big enough to warrant the trouble and expense of introducing a policy or program? The decision should be based on absolute differences in outcomes (population attributable risks), rather than relative risks, since a small effect on a large proportion of the population may be

Box 6-7. Using health data to identify priority risk factors

A report from the Centers for Disease Control and Prevention (1993) illustrates the use of the population attributable fraction to estimate the deaths from several causes that are attributable to a single risk factor. The SAMMEC (smoking-attributable mortality, morbidity and economic cost) computer program was used to estimate the total number of deaths and years of potential life lost attributable to smoking in the United States. For numbers of deaths, the results were as follows:

Neoplasms	179,820
Cardiovascular diseases	148,322
Respiratory diseases	84,475
Infant diseases	1,711
Burns	1,362
Results of environmental tobacco smoke	3,000
TOTAL	418,690

Age-adjusted rates of attributable deaths were also calculated.

The disease impact assessment system (Sainfort and Remington, 1995) described in Box 4-2 illustrates use of the population attributable fraction to estimate the proportion of the burden from a single disease that is attributable to several different risk factors. The program contains relative risks and risk factor prevalence data drawn mainly from the behavioral risk factor surveys for the risk factors of the nine chronic diseases it considers; a community that has its own risk factor prevalence data can insert them. The user inserts population data for the target area, and the program then calculates an estimate of the number of deaths (cases, hospitalizations costs, etc.) from each disease that is attributable to each risk factor. For coronary heart disease, the number of Wisconsin deaths attributable to each risk factor was

Elevated cholesterol	5454
Inactivity	4421
Overweight	4102
Hypertension	3686
Smoking	3191
Diabetes	1726
High-density lipoprotein	1721

Since a person can have more than one risk factor, these figures overlap one another and cannot be added. It is important to remember that this analysis considers only a single cause of death.

Table 6-1. Prioritizing Risk Factors

Risk Factors	Prevalence (p)	Disease A	B	C	Total
1	p_1	Given: RR_{1A} $PAF_{1A} = 1 - (1/\Sigma p_1 RR_{1A})$ $AM_{1A} = PAF_{1A} M_A$	RR_{1B} PAF_{1B} AM_{1B}		ΣAM_1
2	p_2	RR_{2A} PAF_{2A} AM_{2A}			ΣAM_2
3	p_3				ΣAM_3
Mortality (M)		M_A	M_B	M_C	M (all causes)

sufficient to justify a policy. Finally, are the adverse effects of the policy outweighed by its benefits?

The approaches of Laupacis et al. (1992) and Guyatt et al. (1995) provide a mainly economic basis for prioritizing interventions (see Section 5.3), but it is likely that such highly structured approaches can be applied to relatively few policies (as distinct from clinical treatments). A nonquantitative approach based on need and impact was suggested by an Ontario Task Force (Needs/Impact-Based Planning Task Force, 1996:19), summarized in Table 6-2; the eventual decisions would obviously depend upon the way the categories are defined. The Task Force recognized that other factors should also be considered, using the acronym CLEAR: Community capacity, Legality, Efficiency, Acceptability, and Resource availability. Other relevant variables are ethical issues and relevance to societal priorities such as individual responsibility and equity.

Table 6-2. Needs/Impact-Based Planning: When Should an Intervention Be Introduced?

Estimated Impact	Assessed Need High	Medium	Low
Works well	Must do	Must do	Do
Works	Must do	Do	Do
May work	Maybe do/research	Maybe do/research	Research
Does not work	Stop/do not start	Stop/do not start	Stop/do not start

Source: Needs/Impact-Based Planning Committee (1996:19).

A disease model considers more of the relevant factors than any of the above approaches and allows testing of various scenarios, even helping to find the optimal mix when multiple interventions are available (e.g., whatIf? Decision Support Tools, Robbert Associates Ltd., 340 MacLaren Street, Ottawa, Canada K2P 0M6).

Contribution of Public Input to Decision Making

Public policies are made by the public's agents, but it is increasingly believed that direct public input is also required. A substantial social science literature exists on the appropriate role of public input and on the methods for obtaining and using it; this section is included mainly to remind epidemiologists of the importance of public input and to make some preliminary suggestions.

Lomas (1996) observes that the public is not particularly willing to pronounce on many health policy issues and warns that their advice on other issues may not be what policymakers wish to hear. For example, they are inclined to argue for higher expenditures on health care even when governments are desperate to control costs, and are willing to advise ethically questionable limitations on access by various population groups (Bowling, 1996). Many investigators have observed the quite different rankings of interventions produced by the public, such as favoring high technology and acute interventions, and by patients and health professionals, such as favoring supportive services. Jordan et al. (1998) provide a useful categorization of methods for obtaining public input (Table 6-3), according to the extents to which the participants are informed and are given the opportunity to deliberate. An epidemiologist might first consider a survey of the public, but this tends to be expensive, and it is difficult to provide respondents with sufficient information. Social scientists would more likely suggest open forums, calls for written submissions, open telephone lines, key informants, and focus groups, but these qualitative approaches are vulnerable to manipulation by interest groups or domination by vocal individuals. Groups seem to give better advice than individuals, as they benefit from discussion among themselves, and Lomas

Table 6-3. Approaches to Public Consultation on Health Care Priorities

	Informed	Uninformed
Deliberated	Citizens' juries User consultation panels	Focus groups
Undeliberated	Questionnaire surveys with written information	Opinion surveys

Source: Table adapted from Jordan et al. (1998:316).

recommends using panels of 10–20 citizens or patients brought together on a continuing basis to arrive at consensus views, rather than aggregated individual opinions.

Making the Final Decision

Epidemiologic data and methods can help to prioritize problems. But in some cases the necessary data will be lacking. Furthermore, policymakers must address broader issues, e.g., should attention be focused on the short or the long term, on general issues such as efficiency and equity, or on specific health problems like cancer or heart disease? They must also resolve conflicts among the priorities emerging from the earlier methods. The approach to these issues will be influenced by the values and beliefs held by the various players, so the composition of the priority-setting group will be crucial to its results. Epidemiology may be able to influence at least the beliefs through providing a picture of health problems, estimating the associated burden of ill health, modeling health and disease, and advising on the potential effects of focusing on certain areas. But eventually it will be necessary to consolidate the views of the participants. Several of the methods available to assist in this group process have been summarized by the Ontario Task Force (Needs/Impact-Based Planning Committee, 1996), drawn largely from an earlier report (Arthur Young and Company, 1978). They are equally useful for a priority-setting process.

Methods of prioritizing needs or strategies

In the *preference survey method,* no explicit criteria are used. Group members are asked to compare every need or strategy to every other need or strategy, individually assigning a 1 to that considered a higher priority in each dyad, and a zero to that considered a lower priority. The total scores determine the priorities. Internally inconsistent results are possible, e.g., where A is preferred to B, B to C, and C to A.

Social area analysis compares the needs of various geographic areas to the resources available to them. Relevant domains are defined, such as demographic, social, or health status, a weight assigned to each, and one or more indicators identified for each. The areas are then collectively ranked from low to high on each indicator and each area's ranks are summed and averaged within each domain. The average rank is multiplied by the domain's weight and the products are added to produce a summary assessment of need. Resources available to each area are classified as limited, average, or major, and then tabulated against need, to highlight discrepancies.

In the *simplex method* structured questions are developed that can be used to rate health problems on a scale of 1 (lowest priority) to 5 (highest priority), e.g., "Left unattended, this problem is going to (1) get much better; (2) get better; (3) stay the same; (4) get worse; (5) get much worse."

After reviewing all the available information, each member completes the questionnaire independently for each health problem. The average score for each question-alternative combination is calculated across participants, and these values summed across questions to determine the priority to be assigned to each problem. Weights may be assigned to the various questions.

The *Hanlon method* (Hanlon and Pickett, 1984) prioritizes problems or solutions based on four components: size of problem, seriousness of problem, effectiveness of solutions, and PEARL (feasibility) factors. One or more criteria are developed for each of the first three components. Each individual then scores each problem or strategy on each criterion, using a scale from 0 (low) to 10 (high) for size and seriousness, and from 0.5 (problem cannot be resolved at all; strategy will not achieve desired results) through 1.0 (problem can be partly resolved; strategy will just achieve desired result) to 1.5 (problem can be completely resolved; strategy will achieve more than desired result) for effectiveness. The scores are averaged across participants, and then across the criteria for each component, and the results inserted into the following formula:

Basic Priority Rating = (Size + Seriousness) X Effectiveness of Solution

Next, participants consider the PEARL factors: *Political/Public will, Economic feasibility, Acceptability, Resource availability,* and *Legality.*

The question to be answered is: "Do the factors in PEARL permit pursuing solutions (this solution) to the problem?" Each participant rates each alternative on each factor, assigning scores of 1 (yes) or 0 (no) (CLEAR factors could also be used, as listed above). The results are tabulated and discussed, and then the group collectively assigns each alternative a score of 1 or 0 on each factor. The scores for the factors are multiplied together, so that a 0 on any factor produces a 0 PEARL score. The results are incorporated into a second formula:

Overall Priority Rating = Basic Priority Rating X PEARL

Many variations of these approaches exist or can be developed. Box 6-8 presents simplified examples of the output from a participant using each method to prioritize options A, B, and C.

Methods for prioritizing strategies
Moody's precedence chart (Moody 1983:87–111) is identical to the preference survey method, but the Task Force report recommends that participants be asked to use the "best available evidence" (based on a hierarchy of evidence) as the basis for the judgements. Ties in the final scores are resolved by giving preference to the alternative favored in the original one-on-one comparison. Moody (1983) actually presents four variants of the

Box 6-8. Methods to prioritize needs or strategies

Preference Survey

	A	B	C	Total Score
A	xxx	0	1	1
B	1	xxx	1	2
C	0	0	xxx	0

Insert 1 if row preferred, 0 if column preferred.

Social area analysis

Domain	Weight	Indicator	Rankings			Scores		
			A	B	C	A	B	C
Target group	0.3	age	1	3	2	0.3	0.9	0.6
Disease burden	0.7	disability days	2	3	1	1.4	2.1	0.7
TOTAL	1.0					1.7	3.0	1.3

Simplex Method

Question	Options	Rating		
		A	B	C
Affects high-priority group?	1. Other			
	2. Elders			
	3. Women	4	5	1
	4. Disabled			
	5. Children			
Size of resulting burden	1. Very low			
	2. Low			
	3. Medium	2	5	3
	4. High			
	5. Very high			
TOTAL SCORE		6	10	4

Hanlon Method (criteria within domains not shown)

Domain	Range	Rating		
		A	B	C
Size	1–10	3	10	2
Seriousness	1–10	5	9	4
Effectiveness	.5–1.5	1.2	1.5	1.0
Basic priority rating		9.6	28.5	6.0
Feasibility	0 or 1	0	1	1
Overall priority rating		0	28.5	6.0

precedence charts: simple (described here), multiple-input, combined, and extended.

The *nominal group planning method* (Delbecq and Van de Ven, 1971) adds criteria to support the ratings. Six or more people with diverse backgrounds work with a coordinator. Participants independently complete one or more task statement form(s), listing possible strategies and/or criteria for assessing them. Members then take turns contributing one item at a time to a master list for each task, until all items have been recorded. The group discusses and clarifies the lists, without eliminating any items. Individuals then rank-order the N strategies from 1 (least preferred) to N (most preferred), using whichever criteria they choose (alternatively, the group may decide to use a common set of criteria). Each participant's top 10 rankings are then reported to the group, and the ranks are summed across participants. The results are discussed by the group, and then the participants assign overall ratings to their own top 10 items, assigning 100 to the most desirable option. Participants' ratings are summed to determine the priorities of the group.

The *criteria weighting method* also begins by developing criteria for evaluating strategies, but this method weights the criteria. Each individual assigns a value of one (low) to 5 (high) to each criterion, and the average values become the weight for the criterion. Each member evaluates each strategy on each criterion, assigning a score of -10 to $+10$, and the average score is calculated for each strategy-criterion pair. The average scores awarded to each strategy are then multiplied by the corresponding criterion weights to yield a "criterion significance level" for each strategy-criterion pair. These values are summed across criteria, and the sum divided by the number of criteria actually used to rate each strategy, yielding an "average standardized significance level" for each strategy. The process is repeated for each relevant domain of evaluation, and the average standardized significance level of each alternative summed across the domains to achieve a global rating.

The *decision alternative rational evaluation* (DARE) method is a more elaborate alternative to the criteria weighting method. The criteria are ranked individually from least important to most important, and the average rank is determined. A weight of 1.0 is assigned to the least important criterion. Importance weights are then assigned to the other criteria, expressing each weight as a multiple of the weight of the next lower criterion; multiplying the weights together yields an absolute weight for each. These weights are then added and each is divided by the total to yield a relative weight for each criterion. One of the alternative strategies is designated the reference and assigned a score of 1.0 for all criteria, and the others are assigned scores relative to that reference. Average scores are multiplied by the relative criterion weights, negative criteria such as cost or delay are assigned negative signs, and the products are summed to yield the overall priority.

Box 6-9 presents simplified examples of the output of each method as used to prioritize options D, E, and F.

Box 6-9. Methods to prioritize strategies

Moody's Precedence Chart

	D	E	F	Total Score
D	xxx	1	0	1
E	1	xxx	0	1
F	1	1	xxx	2

On the basis of the best available evidence, insert 1 if row preferred, 0 if column preferred.

Nominal group planning (task statement forms not shown)

Alternative	Ranking*	Rating*
D	2	80
E	1	60
F	3	100

*Strategies ranked below 10th would be left blank.

Criteria Weighting (individual criteria not shown)

Domain	Criteria	Weight	Rating D	E	F	Significance level D	E	F
Cost	1	2	+5	−3	+3	+10	−6	+ 6
	2	4	−3	+2	+4	−12	+8	+16
	3	1	NA	−8	+2		−8	+ 2
Total						− 2	−6	+24
Average standardized significance level (ASSL)						− 1	−2	+ 8
Effectiveness	(ASSL)					+ 8	+3	+ 3
Feasibility	(ASSL)					− 3	−3	+ 4
TOTAL SCORE						+ 4	−2	+15

Decision Alternative Rational Evaluation (DARE)

Criterion	Importance Weight	Absolute Weight	Criterion Weight	Rating D	E	F	Score D	E	F
Feasibility	1.0	1.0	0.16	1	2	5	0.16	0.32	0.80
Cost	1.5	1.5	0.24	1	0.2	0.6	−0.24	−0.05	−0.14
Effectiveness	2.5	3.8	0.60	1	0.3	2	0.60	0.18	1.20
TOTAL SCORE		6.3	1.00				0.52	0.45	1.86

These methods are generally used as starting points rather than rigid formulas, and may be adapted and/or combined for use in a specific setting. For example, the Metropolitan Toronto District Health Council combined the simplex tool and PEARL component of the Hanlon method for its priority-setting method.

Summary

When the potential interventions have been identified and assessed, decisions must be made regarding the approaches to be taken. Disease control may be attempted at various levels. The epidemiologist can provide expertise especially on prevention, including the choice between levels and (for primary prevention) between a population and a high-risk approach. It is sometimes useful to use models of the various interventions to determine their potential population impact. Such models can range from simple extrapolations to computerized macrosimulation or microsimulation models, and may focus on a specific disease or on overall population health. Priority setting should use quantitative assessment of needs and interventions to the extent possible; various group methods can be used when quantitative approaches are not possible and to bring factors such as acceptability and feasibility into the process.

Key References

Arthur Young and Company. *Methods for Setting Priorities in Areawide Healthcare Planning.* United States Department of Health, Education and Welfare, 1978

Gunning-Schepers L. The health benefits of prevention: a simulation approach. *Health Policy* 1989;12:1–221.

Morrison AS. *Screening in Chronic Disease,* 2nd ed. New York: Oxford University Press, 1992.

Rose G. *The Strategy of Preventive Medicine.* Oxford: Oxford University Press, 1992.

7

Policy Implementation

Implementation of policy concerns the drafting of legislation or regulations, negotiation of agreements, allocation of resources, and development of direct programs to achieve policy objectives, which in turn involves activities such as staffing and developing operating procedures. It is not a distinct step from policy formulation, but it is part of the same process, and it can even influence policy formulation (Walt, 1994:153–7). Implementation does not occur automatically; indeed, it has been suggested that only about 30% of policies are ever implemented to any meaningful extent. The chances of policy implementation occurring can be improved by development of an implementation strategy, e.g., goal-setting, and consideration of opportunities and barriers (Walt, 1994:177). Epidemiology plays a limited role in this stage of the policy cycle, although it contributes to goal-setting, resource allocation, and information systems.

7.1 Goal Setting

Goal setting emerged as part of the strategic planning movement that followed World War II, first in defense, then in industry, and then in the public sector. In the health sector goal setting has been espoused particularly by the health promotion movement, because of its ability to focus attention on a topic, maintain a sense of direction, guide resource allocation and programming, and measure progress.

Steps in Goal Setting

The task of goal setting is usually assigned to an agency or a task force. Since the success of the effort depends greatly upon the breadth of support in society, it is important that this group be very credible; it should be widely representative of government, the health sector, and the public. Political input should come from the government of the day, the opposition parties (the future government), and the civil service, which will eventually be responsible for implementation. There cannot be too much discussion and consultation.

In general, the process proceeds from the general to the specific. Terminology is inconsistent, and the boundaries between the levels are often ill-defined. Box 7-1 provides examples from the Ontario process of setting goals.

Often the first step is development of a vision statement, which sets out the sort of society toward which the goals will aim, and/or a set of guiding principles or values to which their developers subscribe. Epidemiologists can help in the conceptualization of health and the specification of its determinants; the process is helped tremendously by use of a conceptual framework with a sound theoretical basis.

Box 7-1. Visions, goals, objectives, and targets

The Ontario goals process (Premier's Council on Health Strategy, 1990) included the following components:

- A vision:
  "We see an Ontario in which people live longer in good health, and disease and disability are progressively reduced. We see people empowered to realize their full health potential through a safe, non-violent environment, adequate income, housing, food and education, and a valued role to play in family, work and the community. We see people having equitable access to affordable and appropriate health care regardless of geography, income, age, gender or cultural background. Finally, we see everyone working together to achieve better health for all."

- Five Goals:
  1. Shift the emphasis to health promotion and disease prevention.
  2. Foster strong and supportive families and communities.
  3. Ensure a safe, high-quality physical environment.
  4. Increase the number of years of good health for the citizens of Ontario by reducing illness, disability, and premature death.
  5. Provide accessible, affordable, appropriate health services for all.

- Objectives (one example):
  3.1 Promote individual and community health and well-being by protecting, preserving, and restoring healthy ecosystems.

- Targets (two examples, one nonquantitative, one quantitative):
  3.1.3 Starting immediately, strengthen and accelerate efforts to reduce the environmental impact of energy production and use in Ontario.
  3.1.4 By 2000, reduce by 50% the amount of solid waste being disposed of in Ontario (on a per-capita basis, base year 1987).

The next step is development of a small number of goals: broad statements of desired states or directions in which a society wishes to move. Goals are generally not quantitative and are not necessarily attainable, but they can be very useful as statements against which proposals for policy or program development can be tested. Epidemiologists can advise the goal developers on the feasibility of developing objectives from the proposed goals, but the key input will be from citizens and politicians. Up to this stage, criticism can be expected that the vision is utopian and the goals ill-defined; words like "motherhood" and "warm and fuzzy" will be invoked, but the critics should be reassured by the next stage.

Objectives begin to make the goals realizable. They are more specific and are measurable; therefore they must specify the target population, the intended intervention, and the indicator by which progress will be measured. In short, objectives must be SMART: *S*pecific, *M*easurable, *A*chievable, *R*elevant (to the goals they are supporting), and *T*imed. Normally there will be several objectives for each goal. There is often anxiety about objectives that cannot be quantified: should the process of setting objectives include listing unmeasurable objectives or risk narrowness by omitting them? The answer is surely that objectives should be quantified whenever possible through as much creativity as can be mustered, but one should not hesitate to include objectives that are not currently quantifiable. Epidemiologists can be helpful here, contributing expertise in identification of health indicators and modifiable risk factors.

Targets specify the amount of progress to be made and the time by which it is to be made, allowing more definitive assessments of progress and avoiding later arguments over whether the observed progress constitutes success or failure. Often objectives and targets are combined, as in the United States, where both are called objectives, and in Europe, where both are called targets. This step is essential for subsequent evaluation and is wonderfully exemplified in the United States Mid-Course reviews (Office of Disease Prevention and Health Promotion, 1986), in which graphs indicate the target and trend in the indicator projected to the target year 2000 to allow assessment of whether the goal will likely be met. The role of epidemiology is crucial here: it is important not to invite incredulity by specifying impossible targets or derision by specifying very easy ones. It is equally important to ensure that targets at the various levels be consistent, e.g., that achievement of the targets for risk factor modification would ensure achievement of the targets for disease occurrence. Disease modeling can help in this process; Prevent (Gunning-Schepers, 1989) was developed for this purpose, but the best-implemented example is the use of Can-Trol (Eddy, 1986) in developing the revised cancer objectives for the United States. In the absence of an appropriate disease model, some form of extrapolation will be necessary (see Section 6.2).

Follow-up

The goals will have no impact unless there is substantial support and (especially) action from the many agencies whose activities influence health—achieving this is the hardest step in the process. Equally important, a system must be established to monitor progress toward achievement of the goals, another task for epidemiologists. The momentum of this process in the United States has been impressively maintained under the leadership of the Office of Disease Prevention and Health Promotion. Conversely, health advocates in Ontario failed to obtain adequate support from the civil service, as policy formation tended to ignore the goals process, and from the political opposition, leaving the entire effort to be abandoned when the government changed. Evaluation of progress in achieving the goals and formulation of revised goals again require the services of epidemiologists. Some examples of health goals processes are shown in Box 7-2.

7.2 Allocating Health Resources

Resource allocation is perhaps the most definitive step in policymaking: it is the step in which the money is put where the mouth has been. In principle, the discussion should relate to resources for all programs that influence health, but in practice, given the difficulty in transferring public funds from one sector to another, it usually refers only to funding of public and personal health services. It may be useful to distinguish between *explicit* or *active* resource allocation, in which resources are allocated in advance according to some formula or edict, and *implicit* or *passive* resource allocation, in which things just happen and the allocation can only be described in retrospect. Explicit resource allocation has always been a part of the British National Health Service, so much of the experience in such allocation has been gained there. In non-systems such as in North America, an explicit approach to resource allocation is the exception rather than the rule. With the multitude of payers in the United States, it is difficult to conceive of how a system could operate, except within health maintenance Organizations. In Canada, provincial governments could make explicit resource allocations, but historically they have not; instead, they have simply covered any hospital deficits beyond their defined budgets and paid the bills sent to them by doctors, so the resource allocation could only be recognized in retrospect. This is changing, now that governments are no longer able to pay for everything, and caps and allocations have appeared, although they often seem to be based more on history and ability to pay than on need or expected benefit. Since implicit resource allocation cannot be expected to achieve social goals, this section is about explicit (active) resource allocation. Epidemiologists may be called upon to advise on need, equity, and effectiveness.

Box 7-2. Examples of health goal setting

The process in the United States is highly structured, showing the influence of the management by objectives movement (McGinnis et al., 1997). It has been led by the Office of Disease Prevention and Health Promotion in the Department of Health and Human Services. Great importance is attached to measurability; epidemiologists accordingly play a crucial role. Five goals and ten subgoals were established in 1979 (Department of Health, Education, and Welfare, 1979), along with 15 priority areas for action, and were later elaborated into 226 objectives for 1990 (Department of Health and Human Services, 1980). A mid-course review was released in 1986 (Office of Disease Prevention and Health Promotion, 1986). A new set of 319 objectives for 2000 was released in 1991 (Department of Health and Human Services, 1991), and several progress reports have appeared since then. It is interesting that these are objectives for the nation, not for the federal government: from the outset it was recognized that their achievement would require the participation of a broad range of governments and non-governmental organizations.

The European program grew out of the Alma Ata declaration of 1977 (World Health Organization, 1981a), calling for health for all by the year 2000. Led by the Office of Health Promotion at WHO-EURO in Copenhagen, a set of four goals and 38 targets for Health for All 2000 was released in 1984 (World Health Organization, 1985), and a revision appeared in 1989. The European targets place great emphasis on equity, consistent with their basis in health for all, and on the social determinants of health. They are less technically oriented than those of the U.S., focusing more on values than on measurement, although indicators were identified and progress has been monitored. Member countries were encouraged to develop national health targets consistent with the regional targets, along with plans for their achievement, and many have done so.

The movement has spread outside Europe, with Australia having developed a particularly comprehensive goals project (*Health for All Australians*, 1988); it made very good use of epidemiology in establishing health goals and targets (Leeder, 1995), especially those that were disease-specific. Despite strong encouragement from the Canadian Public Association, Canada has never made more than very tentative moves toward developing national health goals. Several provinces have developed such goals, although not all have continued the process, and several local areas have pursued the approach through public health units or district health councils. Progress made at lower levels will make it more difficult to formulate national goals, should that ever be attempted.

Units of Resource Allocation

To whom or what should health resources be allocated? At least four approaches are possible:

1. *People* (populations). This approach allocates a certain number of dollars to each population group, regardless of their actual utilization. Examples are U.S. health maintenance organizations (although the amount of the "allocation" is determined by the market) and the allocation of health care funding to health regions in the United Kingdom and in some Canadian provinces.
2. *Diseases* or *health problems*. Examples are funding for specialized services for cancer and for mental illnesses. A problem is the susceptibility of this approach to the public appeal of the problem and the political acumen of its supporters.
3. *Providers*. Fixed allocations are made to the hospital sector, physicians, and public health, among others. This has long been the case for highly organized services such as public health and home care and is beginning to happen for hospitals and physicians in the form of budget caps. Such an approach is likely to perpetuate existing patterns of resource allocation, with all their faults, e.g., budget determination by power and history, not by need or efficiency.
4. *Treatments* or *technologies*. Overlapping with the two previous approaches, this one allocates funds to psychotherapy, magnetic resonance imaging, and other treatments. Because of its susceptibility to the political factors noted above, it is unlikely to achieve equity or efficiency in its usual implementation. But allocation of funds to certain "essential services" might be beneficial (see The Case for Defining Essential Services, below).

Basis of Resource Allocation

De Jong and Rutten (1983) describe four principles of resource distribution or allocation. Two principles focus on the *outcome* of resource allocation:

1. *Utilitarianism* is an attempt to maximize the surplus of benefits over costs and thus make the most efficient use of scarce resources. But detailed knowledge of the relation between resources and outcomes is required, and the results may not be fair or equitable. Because the benefits of prevention are long delayed, this approach tends to discourage prevention.
2. *Egalitarianism* is an attempt to equalize the health status within the population as much as possible and thereby achieve equity or fairness. With respect to provision of services, economists refer to *horizontal equity*, in which persons with similar needs are treated similarly, and *vertical equity*, in which persons with different needs are

treated differently, illustrating the relation of egalitarianism with the concept of need. The resulting allocation may not be optimally efficient, although there is empirical evidence that minimizing disparities in health actually improves the overall level of health, as shown, for example, by comparisons of health levels in the United States with those in Japan (Marmot and Davey Smith, 1989), and by the excellent health status of Scandinavian and Dutch populations. Those people in greatest need receive highest priority, but how should need be measured?

Two other principles focus on the *process* of resource allocation:

3. *Equal access* leads to a system that divides resources equally, and thus does not have to measure needs or worry about the effectiveness of services. This principle is therefore very practical and has been adopted by the welfare states, in one form or another. But inasmuch as it ignores the health benefits of the investments made, it may create only the illusion of equity, and may do little to maximize or equalize health.
4. *Libertarianism* is based on the principle of natural rights and simply lets the market work. It is therefore very practical and increasingly espoused by modern politicians, but few thinking persons would claim that it is fair.

Epidemiologists will likely focus on the two outcome-oriented principles and will try to achieve elements of both. De Jong and Rutten (1983) suggest that the egalitarian principle is probably closest to the basic values of most democracies, but that implementation of that principle requires attention to deeper structural features of a society, e.g., public or private ownership of health resources.

Methods of Resource Allocation

"Health resources" refers here to any programs, services, or goods that directly influence health, as well as indirect activities such as income support and environmental protection.

Efficiency-based resource allocation

Following utilitarian principles, this would allocate resources to wherever they would generate preserve or restore the most health. A problem with this type of allocation is that maximum health could be conceivably achieved through allocating additional resources to already advantaged groups, such as lawyers or stockbrokers. This approach requires a metric for health, the most widely advocated being the quality-adjusted life year (QALY). Patrick and Erickson (1993:31) set out a health resource allocation strategy using mainly this approach, with the following steps:

1. Specify the health decision, including the target population, health care alternatives, and assumptions.
2. Classify health outcomes as health states.
3. Assign values to health states.
4. Measure health-related quality of life of the target population.
5. Estimate the prognosis and years of healthy life.
6. Estimate the direct and indirect health care costs under each health care alternative.
7. Rank costs and outcomes of health care alternatives by generating a league table.
8. Revise rankings of costs and outcomes based on stakeholder and community consensus.

The best-known example of the efficiency-based allocation approach is the allocation of Medicaid funding in Oregon (Kitzhaber, 1993), where the government decided that it should fund a narrowed range of effective health services for the whole population, rather than follow the usual pattern of funding a broad range of services (without regard to their effectiveness or efficiency) for one segment of the population (i.e., the poor). Since effectiveness and efficiency of an intervention are peculiar to the condition to which an intervention is applied, it was necessary to define problem-intervention pairs or dyads (cf. needs assessment in Section 4.2) and determine the cost-effectiveness ratio, or the cost of each QALY gained, for each such pairing. They accordingly ranked 709 problem-intervention pairs in decreasing order of QALYs gained or saved per dollar spent (as defined by expert groups) and proposed to begin funding services at the top of the list, proceeding downward until resources ran out. The health care budget of the day was sufficient to cover the target population for 587 problem-intervention pairs. But this rather technical approach produced some apparently nonsensical rankings, such as placing certain dental procedures above life-saving surgery (Eddy [1991] has pointed out that they were not nonsensical at the population level), and was not acceptable to politicians, physicians, or the public (see the third approach for allocating resources). Box 7-3 presents an example of a computer model of efficiency-based resource allocation.

Needs-based resource allocation
Following egalitarian principles, this approach tries to allocate health resources among populations according to their needs. It would seem the most desirable approach in terms of equity, but it raises the question of whether the additional resources will be effective in reversing the disadvantage suffered by some groups. It is also not necessarily efficient. There are many practical problems: How should the population groups be defined? How should the resources be allocated to individuals within groups? This will be a problem unless the groups are quite homogeneous,

---

Box 7-3. The resource allocation framework

A computerized resource allocation framework was devised to support health planning in Ontario in the early 1990s (Angus et al., 1995). The linear-programming model used three types of data: (1) hospital utilization data from the provincial system; (2) cost data from a number of hospitals that were developing disease-costing systems; and (3) estimates of the benefits to be derived from various interventions adapted from the Oregon project. The resulting highly aggregated model was used to estimate the marginal costs and benefits from several scenarios, applied individually and concurrently. These included reducing acute-care beds and lengths of stay, substituting continuing care for acute in-patient care, reducing rate variations and substituting same-day for in-patient surgery, and facility substitution and de-institutionalization. It was concluded that cost savings of about 9% could be realized without significantly compromising the population's health.

---

which implies that they are quite small, but they must be a certain size to average risks sufficiently. Above all, how should need be defined (see Section 4.2) without introducing confounding by current utilization (Birch et al., 1993; Eyles and Birch, 1993)? The best-known example of this approach is the use of the Resource Allocation Working Party (RAWP) formula by the British National Health Service to allocate health care funding to regional health authorities (Department of Health and Social Security, 1976). In the 1970s the RAWP recommended that health care resources be allocated partly according to need, as indicated by the standardized mortality ratio (SMR), and this has been done in one way or another ever since. The SMR has been criticized for saying nothing about the needs of the living, and defended on the grounds that it is not gameable, or capable of being manipulated by an area to increase its allocation, that mortality correlates highly with morbidity, and that a high proportion of health care resources are used just before death. It certainly does not address Culyer's (1992) definition of need, since it ignores capacity to benefit. Many alternative suggestions have been made for specific services, acknowledging that it is not reasonable to expect a single indicator to be appropriate for all types of health care. For example, Eyles et al. (1991) proposed the following combination for determining the allocation of health care resources to a proposed health maintenance organization in Ontario:

- For complications of pregnancy and childbirth: standardized fertility ratio multiplied by standardized very low birthweight ratio

- For in-patient psychiatric services: proportion of the population not married, because of the known correlation of this status with poor mental health.
- For other health care: SMR for persons aged 0–64 by International Statistical Classification of Disease (ICD) chapter.

Allocation according to public preferences

This approach would take the democratic approach of allocating resources to wherever the public wants them allocated. Oregon eventually divided its problem-intervention pairs into 17 broad categories and ranked these groupings at town hall meetings (attended, as it turned out, mainly by health care workers), using the costs per QALY only to rank individual pairs within the groupings (even then, the data were leavened with much expert judgement). One can argue that most resource allocation at present is based on politicians' perceptions of public preferences, but one can also question that assumption, as well as the accuracy of the politicians' perceptions. People are not perfectly informed about cost-effectiveness, are susceptible to various forms of misinformation (witness the results of elections), and are subject to self-interest. And of course, there are many publics. Lomas (1996) has noted that the members of the public serve at various times as taxpayers, collective decision makers, and patients, and that the range of questions on which the public is able and willing to offer opinions is surprisingly narrow:

- as taxpayers, they are able to advise on the overall level of public funding, but not eager to become involved in the details;
- as collective decision makers, they are able (but not very willing) to advise on what broad categories of services should be offered as part of the publicly funded health care system;
- from a patient perspective, they are able (and often very willing) to advise on the socioeconomic circumstances under which patients should be eligible for specific covered services.

See Section 6.3 for methods of obtaining public preferences.

Combining the approaches

It has already been noted that the various approaches may lead to contradictory results. There may be other complications, e.g., the costs of intervention for the same problem may be different in different population groups and in different areas. All three methods seem to have some value, raising the question of how to combine them optimally. It seems reasonable to allocate resources in at least two stages: (1) to defined populations, on the basis of need, and (2) to specific interventions, on the basis of efficiency. As noted above, the Oregon project used public opinion to set broad categories and efficiency criteria within these categories.

The Case for Defining Essential Services

Related to resource allocation is the definition of *essential services,* i.e., those for which health resources must be provided. The Canada Health Act requires the universal health care payment plan to cover all "medically necessary" physicians' and hospital services, but does not define the term explicitly. In The Netherlands, the (Dunning) Government Committee on Choices in Health Care (1992) attempted such a definition. Confronted by scarce resources and no hope of finding more money for health care, and concluding that the scope for increasing efficiency was limited, the committee concluded that society has to make explicit choices regarding what the publicly funded system should cover. It accordingly recommended definition of a list of such services, based on the criteria that such services (1) be necessary to allow every member of society to function normally; (2) be effective; (3) be efficient; and (4) cannot be left to individual responsibility.

Marmor and Boyum (1996) have argued that any attempt to define essential services is simplistic, since the decision on what is essential is not solely technical and the categorization of services as essential or not essential is not binary.

7.3 Information Systems

Too often, information systems are developed for administrative purposes only, without regard to their potential uses for planning and evaluation or for research. Striking examples are the medical care payment plans operated by the governments of the Canadian provinces. When the plans were introduced in the 1960s, epidemiologists pressed the governments to make the system usable for research, surveillance, planning, and evaluation, and particularly to ensure that all the health services received by an individual be identifiable to that individual and hence, linkable. Such a system, if combined with adequate coding of diagnostic and service information, would have permitted the construction of detailed epidemiologic profiles of individuals and the detailed study of utilization of services. This course was taken in Manitoba (Roos et al., 1995) and gradually developed into a comprehensive health information system, which is demonstrating its value (see Section 3.5). But the planners in some other provinces were only interested in paying doctors under the prevailing fee-for-service system and preventing fraudulent billing by them. To maximize the efficiency of collection of premium payments, they enrolled the head of each family as a "subscriber" and registered the other members of the family only when they utilized services. Addresses of the dependents were not recorded, non-utilizers were not registered at all, and errors in recording information about utilizers led to many being listed two or more times. The result is great difficulty in identifying the total utilization of services by an individual and in linking utilization by members of the same family. Planners and evaluators, like researchers, face complex data manipulations before they can use such databases, and are still limited in what can be accomplished. It is likely that those provinces continue to pay a price for their inability to monitor what is happening in their health care systems.

Essential Information To Be Collected

An information system should provide the information needed for policy evaluation and revision. This section addresses the content of such a system (see also Section 8.1 on Evaluating a Current Policy.)

Information required for all policies includes the following:

1. *target population.* This will usually be geographically defined, but for policies directed at subsets of the population, the population meeting the eligibility criteria must be identified (see Section 8.1, Definition of the Target Population). Although it is ideal to list eligible individuals, since this enables linkage to other databases, counts of those individuals, broken down at least by age and sex, will usually be adequate.
2. Key *indicators of implementation,* needed to determine the extent to which the policy was actually implemented. This includes recording key events such as promulgation of legislation or launching of programs, and documentation of what was done compared to what was planned. As in a program evaluation, documentation of implementation is essential for distinguishing a failure of theory from a failure of implementation.
3. *Costs* of the program, including any expenditures from the budgets of other agencies and individuals.
4. Key *outcome indicators,* needed to determine the extent to which the desired outcomes of the policy have occurred (note that this makes no claim regarding the causes of these outcomes, a topic explored in the next chapter). Examples are the proportion of restaurants with designated non-smoking areas, or the prevalence of low birth weight.
5. *Adverse outcomes,* both anticipated, which should be explicitly sought, and unanticipated.
6. *Other events* that might have caused the observed outcomes. Examples are other legislation, media campaigns in neighboring jurisdictions, and pre-existing or concurrent trends. A media clipping service may be an important part of the information system.

Information required for policies that involve the provision of services to *individuals* (i.e., for direct programs) includes the following:

1. Unique *identification of all individuals* in the target population (both users and non-users), along with their age, sex, and residential address

2. All employed or funded *providers,* including their professional qualification (or at least discipline), office address, dates in practice, and
possibly scope of practice
3. All *services provided,* including date of service, unique identification
of provider, unique identification of consumer, reason for encounter
(presenting problem), diagnosis, and services provided (see Sec-
tions 3.5 and 8.3)
4. *Outcomes* (highly desirable but rarely available).

Depending upon the evaluation design (see Section 8.1), it will probably be necessary to collect similar data for other times (before introduction of the policy) or places (which may serve as a comparison group).

Summary

A health goals process assists implementation of policy and enables
evaluation of progress. Goals are general statements defining the situation that is desired, objectives are specific and measurable refinements,
and targets indicate the amount of progress to be achieved and by when.
Epidemiologists can help to ensure that these are realistic, measurable,
and internally consistent. Resource allocation is a key element of implementation and can be oriented to population, problems, providers, or
interventions. The goal of resource allocation can be efficiency (maximizing QALYs per dollar invested) or equity (allocating resources according
to need); the two objective may sometimes be contradictory. Public input
is essential in these decisions. Epidemiology has a role to play in ensuring
that information systems will provide the data needed to support evaluation and revision of a policy.

Key References

Birch S, Eyles J, Hurley J, Hutchison B, Chambers S. A needs-based approach
to resource allocation in health care. *Can Public Policy* 1993; 19:68–85.
McGinnis JM, Harrell JA, Artz LM, Files AA, Maiese DR. Objectives-based
strategies for disease prevention. In: Detels R, Holland WW, McEwen J,
Omenn GS (eds). *Oxford Textbook of Public Health,* Vol. 3, 3rd ed. New York:
Oxford University Press, 1997:1621–31.

8

Policy Evaluation

The choices have been made, the policy implemented, and a reasonable amount of time has elapsed. Has the policy been successful? Strangely enough, its original proponents claim that it has, while its original opponents claim that it has not (perhaps both are right, since they had different objectives for the policy). Can facts be substituted for these opinions? Were the necessary data collected to make that substitution? What information should be collected to prepare for the next cycle?

8.1 Evaluating a Current Policy

Evaluation is "a systematic way of learning from experience and using the lessons learned to improve current activities and promote better planning by careful selection of alternatives for future action" (World Health Organization, 1981b:11). The term encompasses many different approaches, but always implies some sort of judgement regarding the success of an activity. The judgement may be the product of a quick once-over by an expert, a review by the workers involved, or a more formal process. *Systems-oriented evaluation* (Churchman, 1968) looks at a policy or program as a complete organism within its environment and attempts to relate activities and health events in a way that strikes some observers as unsystematic. Epidemiologists are more likely to engage in *goal-oriented evaluation,* which studies the extent to which a policy or program has achieved its objectives. Not surprisingly, this approach is reflected in the definition of evaluation provided by the *Dictionary of Epidemiology* (Last, 1995:57): "A process that attempts to determine as systematically and objectively as possible the relevance, effectiveness, and impact of activities in the light of their objectives." Evaluation always involves consideration of the values of the participants as well as the value of a policy or program.

Dimensions of Evaluation

The evaluation literature refers mainly to programs, but many of the principles and methods are relevant to evaluation of policies. The World Health Organization (WHO; 1981b:16–7) recommends evaluation of six dimensions of health policies and programs, specifying that these dimensions are to be used flexibly:

- *Relevance,* the "response to essential human needs and social and health policies and priorities," essentially their appropriateness
- *Adequacy,* whether "sufficient attention has been paid to certain previously determined courses of action" during problem definition and policy formulation
- *Progress,* monitoring and operational control of ongoing activities during implementation
- *Efficiency* of implementation, the relation between efforts expended and services provided: could the services have been provided more economically? Were they of high quality from a process perspective?
- *Effectiveness,* the degree of attainment of predetermined objectives and targets, with respect to problem reduction or health improvement. This includes community satisfaction and cost-effectiveness of the program (the efficiency of its implementation having been considered under the previous category). It should be quantitative where possible and qualitative where not.
- *Impact,* the overall effect on the health and related socioeconomic development of the target population. Pal (1992:183-93) refers to four types of impact: direct, political, economic, and social. Epidemiologists are equipped to evaluate health impacts, which in the case of health policies are usually direct impacts.

Dunn (1981:343) presents a similar list of six criteria for evaluation:

- *Appropriateness,* or whether desired outcomes are actually worthy or valuable; this criterion resembles relevance
- *Adequacy,* which is similar to the WHO formulation
- *Efficiency,* which is similar to the WHO formulation
- *Effectiveness,* which is similar to the WHO formulation
- *Equity,* or whether cost and benefits are distributed equitably among different groups, is one part of impact (but deserving of special attention)
- *Responsiveness,* or whether policy outcomes satisfy the needs, preferences, or values of particular groups; this criterion seems new and is not particularly related to the WHO's progress. Again, it seems worthy of inclusion.

A simpler approach, developed for quality of care but often applied to evaluation of programs is Donabedian's (1980:79–85) specification of the following evaluative criteria:

- *Structure,* the setting in which care is delivered, including the number and qualifications of staff, organizational structure, and physical facilities

- *Process,* the services provided; this is similar to "progress" in the WHO approach
- *Outcome,* the effects of the service on the client, which is close to effectiveness.

The focus of the Donabedian approach on individual patient–physician encounters accounts for its failure to consider broader factors such as impact on the health of the whole population. It may thus be less applicable to policy.

Dunn (1981:343 ff.) lists three activities that are often called evaluation:

- *Pseudo-evaluation,* which simply measures changes due to the program, without reference to their value or social importance
- *Formal evaluation,* which appears to be identical to goal-oriented evaluation, taking the stated objectives as givens and determining the extent to which a policy has achieved those objectives, normally focusing on effectiveness and efficiency
- *Decision-theoretic evaluation,* which considers the objectives of all the various participants, and examines whether the policy or program is a good idea for society. Thus it addresses all the WHO components and seems most relevant to policy evaluation.

Muir Gray (1997) provides a checklist for assessing a policy evaluation (Box 8-1). Note the (realistic) assumption of a before-after design.

Box 8-1. Criteria for assessing an evaluation of a policy (Muir Gray, 1997:187)

- Were the explicit policy objectives clearly stated?
- Did the research workers identify and articulate any implicit objectives of the policy under investigation?
- Were valid outcome measures identified for each of the explicit and implicit objectives?
- Was data collection complete?
- Were data collected before and after the introduction of the new policy?
- Was the follow-up of sufficient length to allow the effects of policy change to become evident?
- Were any other factors that could have produced the changes (other than the policy) identified in the key criteria and discussed?
- Were possible sources of bias in the research workers acknowledged by the authors or in accompanying editorials?

Determining the Objectives of Policy

The key question in goal-oriented evaluation is whether the policy has been successful in achieving its objectives: "[A] comparison is drawn between actual developments in health status, on the one hand, and the objectives of government policy with respect to public health" (Ruwaard et al. 1994:139). Obviously this requires clear specification of objectives. Such policy objectives should have been stated in advance; if stated after implementation of a policy, it may be tempting to state objectives that have already been achieved, allowing the objectives to be influenced by the outcome. Yet it is remarkable how often the objectives are *not* stated in advance. When the objectives have not been specified, the evaluator's first task to is to identify them through reviewing relevant documents and interviewing key individuals. Often this is not an easy task. When policy involves legislation, its objectives can often be found in the preamble to that legislation.

The persons responsible for developing and implementing the policy must be centrally involved in the statement of objectives to ensure that the important variables are measured and to enhance the probability that they will accept the results. But an evaluation researcher should also be involved to ensure that the objectives are stated in ways that can be measured; objectives are only useful for evaluation if they are measurable. Ideally, a hierarchy of objectives will be developed, including various intermediate changes that are expected to occur as a result of the policy. The objectives should specify the population concerned, the nature of the intervention that is to produce the effect, and the nature of the effect, i.e., the change expected, and the indicators(s) that will measure this. The evaluators may also specify targets, which state the amount of change necessary to warrant calling the policy a success and the time by which the expected change is to be produced. Note the parallel to setting health objectives for a population (Section 7.1), particularly the similarity to SMART objectives. An example of setting objectives is found in Box 8-2.

Definition of the Target Population

The target population of a policy must be defined so that the impact of the policy can be assessed. In principle, it is preferable to identify individuals to permit analysis based on the same, but given the scope and duration of many policies, this is often not practical (see Section 7.3). It is usually acceptable and much more practical to specify only the numbers and characteristics of the target population. When the target is the entire population, as for universal social programs and many environmental control programs, it is readily defined. More often a policy is directed to some segment of the population, and it may then be more difficult to define that segment. Subpopulations may be defined in several ways:

Box 8-2. Promoting heart health in Canada: a focus on cholesterol (Working Group on the Prevention and Control of Cardiovascular Disease, 1992)

An advisory committee to Health and Welfare Canada made a series of recommendations for the control of ischemic heart disease, emphasizing cholesterol control. They specified four "goals" (which look more like objectives):

1. To reduce substantially the number of Canadians at risk from elevated blood cholesterol and other risk factors for ischemic heart disease
2. To reduce the population average blood cholesterol for adult Canadians from the current 5.3 mMol/L to 4.9 mMol/L
3. To reduce average daily intake of total fat and saturated fat to 30% and 10%, respectively of total calories
4. To have Canadian children adopt healthy eating and physical activity habits, maintain a healthy body weight, and avoid smoking.

Supporting these goals were 16 recommendations for strategies to achieve the goals.

- Age, e.g., to measure children's smoking, and/or sex, to study breast cancer prevention, normally present no problem, since population data are readily available.
- Income or education are much more difficult, since data may not exist or may not be available for reasons of privacy protection.
- For most health problems, numbers can be estimated from prevalence data; for cancer it is often possible to identify individuals.
- Groups at particular risk from hazardous exposures or behaviors are yet harder to identify, except for some occupational groups.

Importance of Causal Model

To guide the selection of variables for measurement, it is important to set out a causal model of the way in which the policy or program is expected to work. This can take the form of a *logic model* (Porteous et al., 1997), which lists program components on one dimension and activities, target groups, and short- and long-term outcomes on the other, as shown in Table 8-1. Ultimately, the various cells can be linked by arrows to form a flowchart showing which activities are supposed to produce which effects. It is important to measure key variables at each point in this causal chain to explain why things did or did not work and thereby distinguish a failure of theory from a failure of implementation. The policy or program should not be treated like a black box.

Table 8-1. Logic Model for Evaluating Health Policy

Component	Education	Legislation, regulation	Direct service
Activities	Media	Promulgation, enforcement	Counseling, support
Target groups	Public, professionals	Public	Persons with target disease
Short-term outcomes	Awareness, knowledge	Awareness, compliance	Awareness, utilization
Long-term outcomes	Health behavior change, improved health		

Source: Table adapted from Porteous et al. (1997:4), with permission.

What to Measure

The variables, including relevant intervening variables, and the timing of the measurements need to be specified in advance. As Ruwaard et al. (1994:19) put it, "[r]esearch should also show the extent to which 'attainment' of the calibration points [targets] may be attributed to (government) action taken to that end. For example, in order to be able to evaluate the trend in mortality from lung cancer, besides information on smoking behavior it is also necessary to have data on developments in therapies and on the effect of factors which influence smoking behaviour, such as information, excise measures and legislation covering advertising." Ideally, the information system supporting the policy (Section 7.3) will collect most or all of these variables.

Assessment of implementation will vary with the nature of the policy. Were the regulations passed and promulgated? Did people avail themselves of the benefits, or comply with the regulations? Were the necessary direct programs established and did they reach their target populations?

What health outcomes should be measured? Administrative statistics such as death rates are almost always too insensitive to identify an effect. The same is often true of global measurements of health like the Sickness Impact Profile or the SF-36 (see Section 4.1); in most cases, indicators more specific to the aspects of health targeted by the policy will be needed, e.g., prevalence of specific congenital anomalies at birth, or deaths from burns. Early effects (intermediate outcomes) are particularly desirable indicators, since they may be more sensitive than ultimate outcomes. As always in evaluation, previously validated measures are preferred, if relevant ones can be found.

Sometimes it may not be practical to measure outcomes because they are too long delayed, and then it may be enough to measure the determinants of the outcomes (Ruwaard et al., 1994:33): "Health policy works by influencing determinants. . . The (supposed) effectiveness of health policy can be assessed from improvements in indicators of health status, but also—certainly if a causal relationship is proven—from developments in the determinants of health status (e.g., in risky habits like smoking)."

It is important to monitor potential adverse effects as well as the expected results. Attempts should be made to identify such potential effects in advance, using the literature and expert knowledge. Politicians will also wish to evaluate the costs and the popularity of the policy, but here disciplines other than epidemiology have more to contribute.

When to Evaluate?

Two types of evaluation are usually distinguished in this connection: *formative evaluation,* which conducted during the course of a policy or program, often continually, with a view to improving it; and *summative evaluation,* which is conducted at the end of a policy or program or at some predetermined time to determine whether it has been successful and should be continued.

The timing of a summative evaluation is critical: if it is done too early there may not have been time for the policy to work; if it is done too late, other factors may have intervened that counteracted or overwhelmed its effects. It is common to introduce a policy or program without thought of evaluation and then decide later that it had better be evaluated. This precludes the possibility of "before" measurements and often leads to finding too late that the necessary data have not been collected. It is better to think of evaluation as a continuing process, beginning before the introduction of the policy and continuing throughout its existence. So the appropriate answer to the question of timing is probably "before, during and after," although there may be periodic spurts of heightened activity.

Research Designs for Policy Evaluation

This applies mainly to goal-oriented or "formal" evaluation in which effectiveness is assessed. Did any changes occur in the target variables? If so, were the changes due to the policy or to some other factor (possibly making the policy unnecessary)? Valid answers to these questions depend upon the research design and its ability to isolate the effects of the intervention. It is in the nature of policies that it very difficult to attribute causation: randomization is usually impossible and comparison groups are hard to come by. Various forms of observational studies must therefore be used, ideally quasi-experiments (see Table 5-1), which often offer greater external validity than randomized designs (Campbell and Stanley, 1963) and which may offer the best hope for the assessment of population-level interventions such as policies. In some cases it may be possible to use administrative data for evaluation, bringing the usual advantages of cheapness, large sample size—sometimes the entire population—and (probable) objectivity, counter-balanced by the disadvantage of less-than-perfect relevance. As suggested by the criteria in Box 8-1, the evaluator will often be restricted to a before-after design, which can determine whether a change has occurred, but not the reasons for it (environmental changes, etc.). The design can be improved by providing a basis for predicting what would have occurred in the absence of the policy. This can be achieved by adding a comparison group or by making multiple "before" measures and projecting any trend into the future, turning it into a non-equivalent comparison group or time series design, respectively. Attribution of causation may be strengthened by reference to the flowchart referred to above. Did the expected intervening changes occur in risk factors and determinants? If not, the policy can hardly have been successful. If the expected changes did occur, and if the temporal relationship is correct, this lends some weight to the hypothesis that the policy caused the deviations from the projection. But it will often be difficult to counter the argument that the projection of what would happen in the absence of a policy intervention was simply wrong.

8.2 Monitoring Health Status

This chapter has thus far discussed the evaluation of specific health policies. Another key activity in evaluating (current) policy is observing the health of the population for desirable and undesirable changes. This makes monitoring an important part of the policy process; although it is introduced here, it could also be addressed in Chapter 4 on measuring health status.

Monitoring and Surveillance

The *Dictionary of Epidemiology* (Last, 1995:107) defines monitoring as follows:

1. The performance and analysis of routine measurements, aimed at detecting changes in the environment or health status of populations. Not to be confused with surveillance. To some, monitoring also implies intervention in the light of observed measurements. 2. Continuous measurement of the effect of an intervention on the health status of a population or environment. Not to be confused with surveillance, although the techniques of surveillance may be used in monitoring. The process of collecting and analyzing information about the implementation of a program for the purpose of identifying problems such as noncompliance and taking corrective action.

The first definition recalls debates over whether epidemiology includes interventions to reduce health problems, while the second is directly relevant to evaluation. The closely related concept of surveillance is defined as "[c]ontinuous analysis, interpretation, and feedback of systematically collected data, generally using methods distinguished by their practicality, uniformity, and rapidity rather than by accuracy or completeness" (Last, 1995:163). Despite the warnings not to confuse surveillance with monitoring, the distinction is not clear to everyone and the terms are often used more or less synonymously in practice. It may be useful to think of monitoring as looking for something that is expected (whether a desired outcome or a feared adverse effect), and of surveillance as looking for something unexpected.

Surveillance Systems

Surveillance techniques are relevant here because of their contribution to monitoring. Two books on public health surveillance have appeared from the Centers for Disease Control, one focusing on methods (Teutsch and Churchill, 1994) and the other on applications (Halperin and Baker, 1992), although there is substantial overlap between the two. The CDC's definition of public health surveillance is

> the ongoing, systematic collection, analysis, and interpretation of health data essential to the planning, implementation, and evaluation of public health practice, closely integrated with the timely dissemination of these data to those who need to know. The final link of the surveillance chain is the application of these data to prevention and control. A surveillance system includes a functional capacity for data collection, analysis, and dissemination linked to public health programs (Centers for Disease Control, 1988, cited in Halperin and Baker, 1992:1).

Surveillance can focus on diseases or risk factors as well as the utilization and effects of health services. Quality of surveillance is important in terms of completeness or representativeness of case identification and accuracy of data. An International Working Group for Disease Monitoring and Forecasting (1995) emphasized the need to recognize undercount in surveillance systems, quantify it, and adjust for it using capture–recapture and related methods (see Section 4.2). There is often no need to count every case, only a representative sample.

Components of a surveillance system

Teutsch and Churchill (1994:19) identify the following steps in planning a surveillance system:

1. Establish objectives, indicating which diseases or health problems are to be counted
2. Develop case definitions.
3. Determine the data source or data collection mechanism.
4. Develop the data collection instruments.
5. Field-test the methods.

6. Develop and test the analytic approach.
7. Develop the dissemination mechanism.
8. Assure use of the analysis and interpretation.

Similar steps should be followed by the epidemiologist working on policy, although in this case it is more likely that routinely collected (administrative) data can be used.

Detecting Patterns in Space

This activity can be comparatively straightforward for acute diseases, especially when the background (nonepidemic) incidence is very low, but it is usually much more difficult for chronic diseases, for which the place of occurrence is undefined and the variation in incidence rates much less.

Mapping

It is surprising that mapping has only recently been widely adopted by epidemiologists (except for the traditional spot map of cases of communicable diseases). Most experience in this approach has been gained in preparation of the cancer atlases, which exist for many countries (Walter and Birnie, 1991). Maps can summarize a tremendous amount of information very quickly and make it instantly comprehensible to the reader. They have special meaning for the residents of the area mapped and for their elected politicians. Issues that arise in mapping include those discussed below.

What to map? The location of the occurrence of a disease is most relevant to determining causes and to prevention. In the case of acute injuries, environmental incidents, and occupational and some communicable diseases, location is straightforward and is traditionally plotted on a *spot map*. Potential sources of contamination or infection can be plotted on the same map. A problem with mapping location of events is that the underlying population density, e.g., persons present during working hours, is usually not known, so the denominator is unclear and the pattern hard to assess: a concentration of cases may simply reflect the underlying concentration of people at risk. For most noncommunicable diseases the place and date of occurrence are unknown and usually long past; in these cases only the usual address of the person affected is available. Of course, location of residence is directly relevant to planning services. Addresses can be coded to administrative areas and then simply counted to indicate the absolute burden of illness, or rates or standardized mortality ratios (SMRs) computed for each area.

Choropleth maps present each level or category of such variables coded in a different pattern or color. A major limitation of choropleth maps is their inflexibility: patterns or clusters of health effects do not conform to administrative boundaries and may be obscured when such boundaries are used. The distributions of potential risk factors can be presented as overlays. Geographic information systems have made it possible to code both the location of health events and the distribution of potential causal factors to a very high degree of specificity (Briggs and Elliott, 1995).

Choice of colors. The psychology of perception is important in interpreting a choropleth map, e.g., the colors used, and the intensity of those colors. Gradations of a single color are easiest to interpret; shades of gray are easily interpretable and can be produced on an ordinary laser printer. The choice of categories or cutoffs strongly influences the observed pattern. The Statistical Analysis System (SAS) allows continuous shading, in which depth of color is proportional to the disease rate (Swift, 1993). When mapping SMRs, with their built-in comparison to the reference population, a case can be made for the familiar traffic system of red and yellow for higher than average and green for lower. Maps with no orderly system, e.g., different colors for each category instead of gradations of a single color, are extremely difficult to interpret and should be avoided.

Production of maps. Virtually all maps are now generated by computer, using standard statistical packages or stand-alone programs. Epidemiologists may be most familiar with Epi Map, a relative of Epi Info (USD, Inc., 2075-A West Park Place, Stone Mountain, GA 30087). All these programs require a boundary file to indicate the areas, available from national statistical agencies and from commercial firms. Epi Map provides files for national boundaries for all countries and for counties within the United States.

Limitations. Usually only one variable per map can usefully be presented, using colors or shading. Additional variables soon become confusing; maps are mainly descriptive tools. Maps invite multiple comparisons, with the detection of "patterns" that may be due to chance alone. A large, thinly populated area (perhaps rural or suburban) can dominate a map, overshadowing smaller areas (e.g., cities) where far more people live. Isodemographic maps, which distort boundaries so that the size of each jurisdiction is proportional to its population, can be constructed, but these require specialized techniques and lose some of the immediate relevance that maps have for the reader.

Cluster analysis
Although very striking patterns are identifiable from a map, more often the pattern is less apparent, and some sort of statistical analysis is required. Various methods are available, including quadrat count methods, which divide a region into small areas and count the number of cases in each, and distance methods, which evaluate the distance between cases (Alexander and Boyle, 1996). An inherent problem in evaluating spatial

clustering is the effect of population density: naturally there will be more cases where there are more people. Calculation of rates solves only part of the problem, since the rates for subareas depend on how the areas are defined. By allowing the degree of resolution to be varied, geographical information systems have much greater potential to detect clusters or patterns than does use of administrative boundaries. Bayesian techniques can identify patterns that are not obvious, as strikingly illustrated by Estève et al. (1994:122–40) for several conditions in France.

Detecting Patterns in Time

This refers to the occurrence of all the cases in a defined area over time, without regard to their spatial distribution within that area. The issues in finding the pattern in the midst of the noise differ for acute and chronic diseases.

Acute episodes

Best developed is the investigation of acute outbreaks (Gregg et al., 1996), for which plotting an epidemic curve (number of incident cases against time) may be sufficient. Analysis is usually confined to visual inspection. It is well known that a sharply peaked curve suggests a point source for an outbreak, whereas an extended and irregular pattern suggests person-to-person transmission.

   More relevant here is detection of the excess occurrence of adverse events such as cancer incidence and operative complications. This may be attempted by simple visual inspection, but techniques borrowed from industrial quality control yield more predictable results. Both the following approaches evaluate the number of adverse events occurring during predetermined equal time intervals. The *cumulative sum technique* compares the observed number of events to the expected number, based on prior experience. A reference value K is determined, based on the average number of events per time interval (van Wyck and Hockin, 1984). The cusum statistic Q is initially set at zero and replaced at the end of each time interval by the larger of 0 and the sum of the current Q plus the difference between the number of events X during the interval and K:

$$Qt = \max [0, (Qt_{-1} + Xt - K)]$$

Thus, Q can increase or decrease, but it can never become negative. A warning signal is raised whenever Q exceeds some preset threshold, chosen to balance the numbers of false positives and false negatives. Box 8-3 illustrates a potential application of this technique.

   Hill (1983) adapted the technique for use in a cancer registry, in conjunction with exponentially weighted moving averages. The expected number of events in each interval is calculated using the formula

$$Et = Et_{-1} + A(Ot_{-1} - Et_{-1})$$

where E is the expected and O the observed number of events, and A is an empirically derived constant. A standardized score X is then calculated for each interval:

$$Xt = \frac{Ot - Et}{\sqrt{Et}}$$

and used in the formula for cusum.

The *scan statistic* considers the maximum number of events occurring in a series of equal predetermined time intervals (Stroup, 1994). Published tables or computer simulations provide the probability that the maximum number of events will equal or exceed the observed value, based on the total number of events and the number of intervals. With any such approach, the risk of false alarms is real, and the challenge is to adjust the system to yield adequate sensitivity at tolerable levels of specificity. More sophisticated approaches are available (Stroup and Thacker, 1993).

Long-term trends

For most noncommunicable diseases clusters are not usually an issue, and the pattern is a complex of seasonal variations and *secular trends*. A *secular trend* is a long-term systematic change in age-specific rates over calendar time (Kleinbaum et al., 1982:132). The simplest technique for detecting trends is simple linear regression of disease rates or some transformation thereof on time. More elaborate analyses include ARIMA (autoregressive integrated moving average) models (see Section 4.4). A secular trend can be explained by the effects of (calendar) period, birth cohort, or some combination of these. These concepts can be summarized in a Lexis

---

Box 8-3. Early detection of an outbreak

In the early 1980s an excess of deaths was noted among postoperative cardiac surgery patients at a pediatric hospital (Buehler et al., 1985). By the time the excess was recognized, over 30 infants had died. Subsequently, an epidemiologist entered the data into a computer programmed to compute cusum, and found that the alarm rang after fewer than 5 deaths. If the hospital had had such a program in place, could the remaining deaths have been avoided? Or is this just the wisdom of hindsight? If the program were in place, what could have been done about the inevitable false alarms?

diagram (see Figure 8-1), in which person-time (age) is plotted against calendar time. The diagonal dotted lines indicate the experience of birth cohorts, with some untidiness resulting from the overlap of the diagonal paths on the corners of adjacent squares.

Traditionally, graphical *cohort analysis* has been used to disentangle these effects, usually by plotting the age pattern of mortality by birth cohorts, rather than the more conventional periods of death, to display the lifetime experience of each birth cohort. More recently, statistical *age–period–cohort analysis* has become widely used (Kupper et al., 1985; Holford, 1991). Results emerge in the form of regression coefficients or relative risks for each component of the trend. Such analyses are plagued by the *identifiability problem*: the three effects are not independent, so if any two are known, the third can be calculated. The result is that there is always an alternative explanation for any finding; e.g., an apparent cohort effect can be equally well explained as a combined age and period effect.

8.3 Monitoring Health Care Utilization

Measuring Health Care

Chapter 3 discussed the availability of data for health care utilization. Here we discuss their manipulation and interpretation. Only hospital and physicians' services data are sufficiently available and consistent to war-

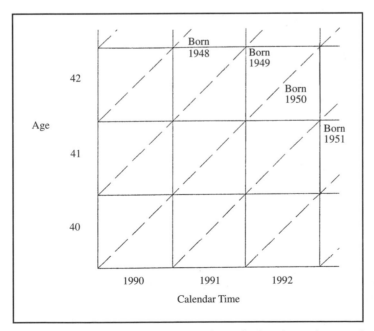

Figure 8-1. Lexis diagram. Diagonal lines indicate birth cohorts, born in the years indicated. Thus persons born in 1950 turn 40 in 1990, 41 in 1991, etc.

rant consideration here, but the principles apply to most other services. Denominator issues become important when utilization of specific providers is considered, whereas numerator issues concern units of analysis.

Hospitals
Catchment population.
The catchment population of any service includes both users and nonusers of the service, and both must be identified and monitored: it is not enough to count users. In many health care systems, the catchment populations of hospitals are not defined, and there is considerable flow of patients across geographic boundaries. It is therefore necessary to make some estimate of the catchment or referral population for a specific hospital or group of hospitals. A common empirical approach (describing where patients go, as distinct from where health planners think they should go) is to generate something like Table 8-2, where H_{1A} is the hospitalization experience (either separations or days of care) of members of population 1 in hospital A, ΣH_1 is the total hospital experience of population 1, and CP_A is the catchment population for hospital A; note that ΣCP equals the total population, ΣP. The bed supply is calculated as follows:

$$\text{Bed Supply Ratio} = \frac{\text{Beds}}{\text{Catchment Population}}$$

An alternative approach (Roos, 1993) uses the admitting practices of the referring physicians.

Hospital utilization. The term *separation* includes all the ways that a patient can leave hospital: discharge, walk-out, transfer, and death. It is sometimes preferred to "admission" because the latter does not include births (newborns are not separately admitted to hospital). Inasmuch as admissions and separations are events, they can be treated in the same way as incidence (in the case of one-time conditions that are always hospitalized, such as appendicitis, they may be a reasonable surrogate for the incidence of disease):

$$\text{Separation Rate} = \frac{\text{Number of Separations}}{\text{Person-Time}}$$

For stable annual rates, this approximately equals the number of separations divided by the catchment population.

Total *days of care* are another widely available statistic for hospital utilization. They also lend themselves to calculation of rates, so that

$$\text{Days of Care Rate} = \frac{\text{Total Days of Care}}{\text{Person-Time}}$$

Table 8-2. Calculating Hospital Catchment Populations

	Population	Hospital A	Hospital B	Hospital C	Total
Region 1	P_1	$CP_{1A} = (H_{1A}/\Sigma H_1) \times P_1$	$CP_{1B} =$	$CP_{1C} =$	ΣH_1
Region 2	P_2	$CP_{2A} =$	$CP_{2B} =$	$CP_{2C} =$	ΣH_2
Region 3	P_3	$CP_{3A} =$	$CP_{3B} =$	$CP_{3C} =$	ΣH_3
TOTAL	ΣP	ΣCP_A	ΣCP_B	ΣCP_C	ΣH

Days of care are related to the *prevalence of hospitalization*, which equals the average proportion of the population that is in hospital on any given day:

$$\text{Prevalence of Hospitalization} = \frac{\text{Days of Care Rate}}{365}$$

Average length of stay is analogous to the duration of an illness, and can be calculated from the basic epidemiologic equation relating prevalence and incidence:

$$\text{Average length of stay} = \frac{\text{Days of Care}}{\text{Separations}} \approx \frac{\text{Days of Care Rate}}{\text{Separation Rate}}$$

The steady-state assumption is especially important here, given the frequency with which these parameters change.

Occupancy "rates" (really proportions) reflect the extent to which available beds are used. Bearing in mind that a hospital bed is available for 365 days per year,

$$\text{Occupancy} = \frac{\text{Days of Care}}{\text{Operating Beds} \times 365}$$

Finally note that:

$$\text{Prevalence of Hospitalization} = \text{Bed Supply Ratio} \times \text{Occupancy}$$

Examples of the calculation of these indicators are found in Box 8-4.

Physicians

Denominator issues. For whose care is a physician responsible? This question has been addressed mainly in primary care research, but similar

---

Box 8-4. Indicators of health care

Carrying out the calculation in Table 8-2 for acute care (excluding new-borns, acute psychiatric care, and care for non-Ontario residents) provided by the hospitals in the Regional Municipality of Ottawa-Carleton yielded a catchment population of 837,017 (Health Services Restructuring Commission, 1997) in 1994-95. It is not surprising that this total is considerably larger than the Ottawa-Carleton population of 736,156, since Ottawa is a referral center.

Given that there were 1878 acute beds in Ottawa-Carleton in 1995–96, the bed supply ratio was 1878/837,017 = 0.00224 or 2.24 beds per 1000 population (ignoring the discrepancy in year).

There were 78,347 separations in 1995–96, for a separation rate of 78,347/837,017 = 0.0936/year or 93.6 separations per 1000 person-years.

A total of 536,667 days of care were provided, so the days of care rate was 536,667/837,017 = 0.641/year or 641 days per 1000 person-years.

The average length of stay was 536,667/78,347 = 6.85 days (calculated from rates, 641/93.6 = 6.85 days).

The average occupancy was $536,667/(1878 \times 365) = 0.783$ or 78.3%.

The average prevalence of hospitalization (proportion of the population that was in hospital at any one time) was $0.641/365 = .00224 \times 0.783 = .00175$, so on average, 1.75 of every 1000 members of the catchment population were in hospital on any given day.

---

methods are applicable to other health services. Several approaches to defining the catchment populations are possible:

1. *Geographical definitions* may be adequate in isolated areas where patients have access to only one physician or group practice.
2. *Rosters* (lists) are of two types (Spitzer et al., 1978):
a. *Registry-derived rosters* are lists of persons who have designated a certain practice as their source of primary medical care, as happens automatically with the capitation method of paying physicians.
b. *Utilization-derived rosters* are based upon what people do, as distinct from what they say they will do. They require an arbitrary definition, e.g., the practice at which an individual obtains at least one half (or two-thirds, or more than anywhere else) of her care. Most utilization-based rosters ignore non-users. It is also possible to distribute patients among physicians as was done for hospitals (above).
3. *Projections from users* include the following two models:
a. *Proration.* If it is known that 70% of a population visits a primary care physician during a year, then the denominator for a given practice can be estimated by dividing the number of different persons

who actually visit during a year by 0.70. Obviously, this assumes that utilization patterns, accessibility, and other factors, are the same in this practice as the average for the entire population, which is a large assumption.

b. *Mathematical modeling.* Kilpatrick (1975) demonstrated that the frequency distribution of visits per year in many British practices fit the negative binomial distribution remarkably well. Having estimated the parameters for a practice from the utilizers, he used the distribution to estimate the number of individuals who made zero visits to the practice. Unfortunately, the approach worked much less well in North America (Cherkin et al., 1982).

Numerator issues. The key decision in measuring utilization of physicians' services is determining the units, for which there are several possibilities, none of them ideal. Their availability depends largely upon the payment mechanisms for physicians:

- Visits are usually feasible under fee-for-service remuneration, but vary widely in their content and are subject to wide variations in practice and billing patterns.
- Services are a loosely defined concept dependent entirely upon the fee schedule in use; e.g., a hysterectomy and a visit for an allergy injection may each count as a single service.
- Fees (payments) may provide a better idea of the intensity of the medical care received, but are also subject to the peculiarities of fee schedules (see Economic Burden of Ill Health, Section 4.1);
- Episodes of care provide a closer approximation to incidence of morbidity and avoid distortions due to practice patterns, but are notoriously hard to define.

Small-Area Variations in Health Care

Comparisons of small areas are useful for determining areas of special need, such as inequalities in health and specific local hazards, and for assessing how well the health system is working. The former has been addressed in the section on small-area estimates in Section 4.1. The latter was developed initially by Wennberg and Gittelsohn (1982), who discovered puzzling disparities in the rates of medical care, especially surgical operations, which are easy to count, within various areas of New England. Similar differences have been found in many other areas (Roos and Roos, 1981; Goel et al., 1996). Indeed, marked variations in this important aspect of physician behavior seem to be the norm rather than the exception, and epidemiologists need to know how to identify and interpret them.

Methods for detecting variations

The challenge is to define the areas to be studied so that they are large enough to be stable, but small enough not to average out any variation.

Cities or counties are the choice in most cases. In the following section, Y_{ij} refers to the number of procedures provided to person j in area i per year. If there are no repeat procedures (as for organ removal, such as cholecystectomy), Y_{ij} equals 0 or 1 and the area mean ($\bar{Y}_i$) equals the proportion of individuals who receive the procedure (cumulative incidence over 1year) in area i. When multiple procedures or admissions are possible, it is necessary to introduce a *multiple admission factor* (Diehr et al., 1993). Several indicators are used to express the results, the choice having to do with whether an indicator accounts for within-area (random) variation, the overall incidence of the procedure (issue of absolute versus relative differences), and the varying sizes of the areas (Diehr et al. 1993).

Extremal quotient (EQ). The EQ is the ratio of the largest to the smallest mean value:

$$E\,Q = \frac{\overline{Y}_{max}}{\overline{Y}_{min}}$$

Its value depends upon the way the areas are defined; it is determined only by the extreme values, which usually belong to areas with very small populations. Furthermore, the EQ does not reflect the overall frequency of the procedures. Indeed, the EQ appears to have no redeeming qualities.

Coefficient of variation (CV). The CV is the ratio of the standard deviation of the area means to the overall mean. This measure obviously adjusts for the overall frequency of the procedure, but in its first two versions it ignores within-area variation. The unweighted version gives equal weights to all regions, regardless of their populations, and thus treats the area means as equal entities:

$$\text{CV (unweighted)} = \frac{Su}{\overline{Y}u} \; ; \; S^2u = \frac{\Sigma(\overline{Y}i - \overline{Y}u)^2}{k-1}, \; \overline{Y}u = \frac{\Sigma \overline{Y}i}{k}$$

where $\overline{Y}u$ is the unweighted mean of the area means and k the number of areas. The more common (and more reasonable) weighted version gives greater weight to more populous regions:

$$\text{CV (weighted)} = \frac{S_w}{\hat{\mu}} \; ;$$

$$S^2w = \frac{\Sigma[ni(\overline{Y}i - \overline{Y}.)^2]}{(\Sigma ni) - 1}, \; \hat{\mu} = \overline{Y}. = \frac{\Sigma ni \overline{Y}i}{\Sigma ni}$$

where ni is the population of area i and $\hat{\mu}$ (estimated by $\overline{Y}.$) the grand or overall mean. The CV can also be calculated from an ANOVA; then it has the advantages of removing within-area variation, adjusting for multiple admissions, and providing a confidence interval:

$$CV (ANOVA) = \frac{\hat{\sigma}A}{\hat{\mu}};$$

$$\hat{\sigma}A = \sqrt{\frac{MSA - MSW}{n_0}}; \quad n_0 = \bar{n} - \frac{s\hat{n}}{k\bar{n}}$$

where MSA and MSW are the mean squares among and within areas, and $\bar{n}$ and $s\hat{n}$ are the mean and variance of the populations of the areas. Diehr et al. (1993) show that it can also be estimated from chi-square and the multiple admission factor.

Systematic component of variation (SCV). The SCV (McPherson et al., 1982) is unweighted with respect to area population, but adjusts for the frequency of the procedure and removes the within-region variation (provided that there are no repeat procedures). It thereby attempts to express the true variation among regions:

$$SCV = \frac{1}{k}\left[\Sigma\left(\frac{Oi - Ei}{Ei}\right)^2 - \Sigma\frac{1}{Ei}\right]$$

where Oi and Ei are the observed and expected numbers of procedures in area i, the latter calculated on an age- and sex-specific basis.

Chi-square. This indicator is the only standard indicator that provides a statistical test, but its value conveys no meaning in itself:

$$Chi\text{-}square = \Sigma \frac{(Oi - Ei)^2}{E_i}, \quad df = k - 1$$

when the frequency of the procedures is low. It has the disadvantage of being highly statistically significant in virtually every case, and thus lacks specificity.

More elaborate analyses are possible, such as Poisson regression, hierarchical regression, and empirical Bayes estimation, but these are less accessible to non-experts. Diehr et al. (1993) recommend using the CV calculated from ANOVA when the procedures are common and the expected number of procedures in the smallest area is one or more.

Potential explanations
Small-area variations are important because of what they may tell us about the quality and efficiency of care. But several interpretations are possible.

1. Variations in need for services. Variations in utilization rates can only be interpreted if accompanied by information on possible variations in need. In fact, variations in need are rarely found to explain the differences in utilization, suggesting that other factors are at work.
2. Variations in supply of health resources. There is abundant evidence that more beds mean more hospitalizations, more surgeons mean more operations, etc. (see Availability Effect, Section 3.4). But this factor does not explain the whole story.
3. Variations in ability to pay. It is reasonable to expect that people who are able to pay for services would have higher utilization rates than those who are not, but small-area variations are regularly found in Canada, where the direct patient cost for care is zero.
4. Variations in habits, local medical cultures. Physicians in an area can develop characteristic practice patterns, perhaps in response to influential local physicians.
5. Clinical uncertainty. It is widely accepted that conflicting scientific evidence and the lack of clear clinical guidelines can lead to variations in practice behavior, perhaps leaving more room for the other factors to affect variation.
6. Artefact. The usual suspects apply here, the first being *chance*. Interpretation of small-area variations is a classic case of post hoc hypothesis testing—one attempt to assess the probability that something happened after it has happened (in fact, the role of chance is rarely assessed at all). Furthermore, the sampling distributions of the first three of the described statistics are unknown, making statistical testing difficult. As a result, the role of chance in producing small-area variations is too often ignored. Another source of error is *bias*. Variations in utilization rates could conceivably be due to variations in data quality, such as incorrect recording of address, or different methods of counting procedures, but the variations exist when bias is known to be absent. The last possibility is *confounding*. Variations could be explained by differences in age, sex, education, etc., but are frequently found to persist after adjustment for such variables.

The results of a small-area variations analysis are shown in Box 8-5.

Access to Care

Access is an important concept in health services, with relevance to equity and the impact on population. This concept was defined by Aday et al. (1980:26) as "those dimensions which describe the potential and actual entry of a given population to the health care delivery system." Aday

---

Box 8-5. Small area variations in health care

The Practice Atlas, published by the Institute for Clinical Evaluative Sciences (Goel et al., 1996), studied practice variations across Ontario's 33 District Health Councils, using the four indicators referred to in the text. Some sample results follow:

Procedures	Cholecystectomy	Hip replacement
Provincial rate/100,000	339.4	81.5
Extremal quotient	1.9	1.6
Coefficient of variation (weighted)	12.5	11.8
Systematic component of variance	23.0	7.6
Adjusted chi-square (32 df)	416.2	93.0

As expected, all the indicators show greater variability for cholecystectomy (for which the indications are rather uncertain) than for hip replacement (for which the indications are quite clear).

---

et al. (1980:35) distinguish between potential access and realized access in a conceptual framework summarized in Figure 8-2. Most of the suggested indicators have been treated in Chapters 3 and 4. An alternative conceptualization is that of Penchansky and Thomas (1981), who identified five components of access as the "five A's":

- Availability: supply of health care providers in an area
- Accessibility: hours of operation, travel distance, etc.
- Affordability: presence or absence of financial barriers
- Acceptability: sex of providers, cultural sensitivity, language, etc.
- Accommodation: location, physical plant, presence or absence of physical barriers.

In Aday's terms, the first component is a structural indicator of potential access and the other four are all subjective indicators of realized access.

The Wheel Turns

This brings us to the end of the policy cycle; the emphasis on monitoring developments in health portends the next cycle, beginning with the reassessment of health needs.

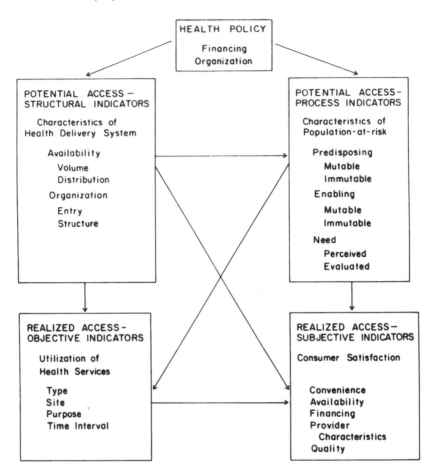

Figure 8-2. Framework for the study of access. [Reprinted from Aday LA, Andersen R, Fleming GV. Health Care in the US: Equitable for Whom? Figure 1-1, page 35, copyright © 1980 by Sage Publications, Inc. Reprinted by permission of Sage Publications, Inc.]

Summary

Evaluation of both policies and programs must be conducted. Epidemiologists can help to state objectives in measurable ways, develop the evaluation design, and provide special expertise in measuring health impact. The objectives of the policy should be clearly stated, and a flowchart or logic model should be constructed to illustrate how it will work. The evaluation design should provide the best possible comparisons of what happened to what would have happened in the absence of the policy. Comparison groups will rarely be feasible (much less randomized control groups), and some sort of extrapolation or modeling may offer the best comparisons possible. It is important to measure variables representing process as well as outcome. In addition to specific evaluations, it is necessary to monitor the health of the population to detect trends and patterns, and especially emerging problems. Monitoring is the process of observing the health status of a population over time. Surveillance is the systematic collection and analysis of information regarding a specific health issue and its dissemination to decision makers. Both are crucial activities for support of health policy—the former to evaluate policies and programs and the latter to identify needs and trends. Maps help to identify spatial patterns and clusters, while Bayesian methods can add analytical power. Techniques borrowed from the quality control literature can help to identify temporal clusters. Time trends can be studied by techniques ranging from relatively simple graphical approaches, such as cohort analysis, to sophisticated statistical analyses, such as age-period-cohort analysis and ARIMA models. Utilization of health services can be measured using methods similar to those used for disease. Small-area variations in health care are ubiquitous, and several methods are available for their analysis. *Access* to care can be assessed indirectly from several types of data.

Key References

Diehr P, Cain K, Ye Z, Abdul-Salam F. Small-area variation statistics: methods for comparing several DRGs. *Med Care* 1993;31(Suppl):YS45–YS53.

Teutsch SM, Churchill RE. *Principles and Practice of Public Health Surveillance.* New York: Oxford University Press, 1994.

World Health Organization. *Health Programme Evaluation: Guiding Principles for its Application in the Managerial Process for National Health Development.* Geneva: World Health Organization, Health for All Series No. 6, 1981.

References

Abramson J. *Survey Methods in Community Medicine: an Introduction to Epidemiological and Evaluative Studies,* 3rd ed. Edinburgh: Churchill Livingstone, 1984.

Aday LA, Andersen R, Fleming GV. *Health Care in the US: Equitable for Whom?* Beverly Hills, CA: Sage Publications, 1980.

Aickin M, Dunn CN, Flood TJ. Estimation of population denominators for public health studies at the tract, gender and age-specific level. *Am J Public Health* 1991;81:918–20.

Alexander FE, Boyle P (eds). *Methods for Investigating Localized Clustering of Disease. IARC Sci Publ* 1996;135.

Altman DG, Balcazar FE, Fawcett SB, Seekins T, Young JO. *Public Health Advocacy. Creating community change to improve health.* Palo Alto, CA: Stanford Center for Research in Disease Prevention, 1994.

American Psychiatric Association. *Diagnostic and Statistical Manual of Mental Disorders* (DSM), 4th ed. Washington, DC: American Psychiatric Association, 1994.

Angus DE, Auer LO, Cloutier JE, Albert T. *Sustainable Health Care for Canada.* Queen's-University of Ottawa Economic Projects. Ottawa: University of Ottawa, 1995.

Armenian HK, Shapiro S (eds). *Epidemiology and Health Services.* New York: Oxford University Press, 1998.

Arrow KJ. *Social Choice and Individual Values,* 2nd ed. New York: John Wiley & Sons, 1970.

Arthur Young and Company. *Methods for Setting Priorities in Areawide Healthcare Planning.* Washington, DC: United States Department of Health, Education and Welfare, 1978.

Balkau B, Jougla E, Papoz L, Eurodiab Subarea C Study Group. European study of the certification and coding of causes of death of six clinical case histories of diabetic patients. *Int J Epidemiol* 1993;22:116–26.

Band PR, Gaudette LA, Hill GB, Holowaty EJ, Huchcroft SA, Johnston BM, Makomaski Illing EM, Mao Y, Semenciw RM. *The Making of the Canadian Cancer Registry: Cancer Incidence in Canada and its Regions, 1969–1988.* Ottawa: Minister of Supply and Services Canada, 1993 (Catalogue Number C52-42/1992).

Barendregt JJ, Bonneux L, van der Maas PJ. The health care costs of smoking. *N Engl J Med* 1997;337:1052–7.

Barker C. *The Health Policy Process*. London: Sage Publications, 1996.

Beaglehole R, Bonita R, Kjellstrom T. *Basic Epidemiology*. Geneva: World Health Organization, 1993.

Bergner M, Bobbitt RA, Carter WB, Gilson BS. The Sickness Impact Profile: development and final revision of a health status measure. *Med Care* 1981; 19:787–805.

Birch S, Eyles J, Hurley J, Hutchison B, Chambers S. A needs-based approach to resource allocation in health care. *Can Public Policy* 1993; 19:68–85.

Bonneux L, Barendregt JJ, Looman CWN, van der Maas PJ. Diverging trends in colorectal cancer morbidity and mortality: earlier diagnosis comes at price. *Eur J Cancer* 1995;31A:1665–71.

Bonneux L, Barendregt JJ, Nusselder WJ, van der Maas PJ. Preventing fatal diseases increases healthcare costs. *BMJ* 1998;316:26–9.

Bowling A. Health care rationing: the public's debate. *BMJ* 1996;312:670–4.

Boyle MH, Furlong W, Feeny D, Torrance GW, Hatcher J. Reliability of Health Utilities Index—Mark III used in the 1991 cycle 6 Canadian General Social Survey Health Questionnaire. *Qual Life Res* 1995;4:249–57.

Braybrooke D, Lindblom CE. *A Strategy of Decision: Policy Evaluation as a Social Process*. New York: The Free Press, 1963.

Briggs DJ, Elliott P. The use of geographical information systems in studies on environment and health. *World Health Stat Q* 1995;48:85–93.

Brownson RC. Epidemiology: the foundation of public health. In: Brownson RC, Petitti DB (eds). *Applied Epidemiology: Theory to Practice*. New York: Oxford University Press, 1998:3–34.

Brownson RC, Petitti DB (eds). *Applied Epidemiology: Theory to Practice*. New York: Oxford University Press, 1998.

Buehler JW, Smith LF, Wallace EM, Heath CW, Kusiak R, Herndon JL. Unexplained deaths in a children's hospital: an epidemiologic assessment. *N Engl J Med* 1985;313:211–6.

Campbell DT, Stanley J. *Experimental and Quasi-experimental Designs for Research*. Englewood Cliffs, NJ: Prentice-Hall, 1963.

Canadian Task Force on the Periodic Health Examination. *The Canadian Guide to Clinical Preventive Health Care*. Ottawa: Health Canada, 1994.

Cartwright A. *Health Surveys in Practice and in Potential: A Critical Review of Their Scope and Methods*. London: King Edward's Hospital Fund for London, 1983.

Centers for Disease Control (CDC). *CDC Surveillance Update*. Atlanta: CDC, 1988.

Centers for Disease Control and Prevention. Cigarette smoking attributable mortality and years of potential life lost—United States, 1990. *Mortal Morbid Week Rep* 1993;42:645–9.

Chambers LW, Woodward CA, Dok CM. *Guide to Health Needs Assessment: A Critique of Available Sources of Health and Health Care Information*, revised ed. Ottawa: Canadian Public Health Association, 1983.

Cherkin DC, Berg AO, Phillips WR. In search of a solution to the primary care denominator problem. *J Fam Pract* 1982;14:301–9.

Chiang CL. *The Life Table and Its Applications*. Malabar FL: Robert E Krieger, 1984.

Chiang CL. Competing risks in mortality analysis. *Annu Rev Public Health* 1991;12:281–307.

Churchman CW. *The Systems Approach*. New York: Dell, 1968.

Clarke EA, Marrett LD, Kreiger N. *Twenty Years of Cancer Incidence 1964–1983: The Ontario Cancer Registry*. Toronto: The Ontario Cancer Treatment and Research Foundation, 1987.

Coale AJ, Demeny P. *Regional Model Life Tables and Stable Populations*. Princeton: Princeton University Press, 1966.

Cochrane AL. *Effectiveness and Efficiency: Random Reflections on Health Services*. The Nuffield Provincial Hospitals Trust, 1972.

Cohen MM, MacWilliam L. Measuring the health of the population. *Med Care* 1995;33(Suppl):DS21–DS42.

Commission of Inquiry. *Public Health in England: The Report of the Commission of Inquiry into the Future Development of the Public Health Function* (Acheson report). Cmnd 289. London: HMSO, 1988.

Coughlin SS. Ban on policy recommendations in epidemiologic research papers? Surely, you jest. *Epidemiology* 1994;5:257–8.

Coughlin SS, Beauchamp TL (eds). *Ethics and Epidemiology*. New York: Oxford University Press, 1996.

Council for International Organizations of Medical Sciences. *International Guidelines for Ethical Review of Epidemiological Studies*. Geneva: CIOMS, 1991.

Culyer AJ. *Equity in Health Care Policy. A Discussion Paper*. Toronto: Premier's Council on Health, Well-Being and Social Justice, 1992.

Dan BB. Dealing with the public and the media. In: Gregg MB, Dicker RC, Goodman RA (eds). *Field Epidemiology*. New York: Oxford University Press, 1996:181–93.

Davey Smith G, Bartley M, Blane D. The Black report on socioeconomic inequalities in health 10 years on. *BMJ* 1990;301:373–7.

DeFriese G (ed). Proceedings of National Research Conference on personal health risk assessment methods in health hazard/health risk appraisal. *Health Services Res* 1987;22:441–620.

DeFriese GH, Fielding JE. Health risk appraisal in the 1990s: opportunities, challenges, and expectations. *Annu Rev Public Health* 1990; 11:401–18.

de Jong GA, Rutten FFH. Justice and health for all. *Soc Sci Med* 1983; 17:1085–95.

Delbecq Al, Veen AH Van de. A group process model for problem identification and program planning. *J Appl Behav Sci* 1971;7:4.

Department of Clinical Epidemiology and Biostatistics. How to read clinical journals. I. Why to read them and how to start reading them critically. *Can Med Assoc J* 1981;124:555–90, and articles in several following issues.

Department of Health and Human Services, Public Health Service. *Promoting Health, Preventing Disease. Objectives for the Nation*. Atlanta: Centers for Disease Control, 1980.

Department of Health and Human Services. *Healthy People 2000: National*

Health Promotion and Disease Prevention Objectives. Washington, DC: Department of Health and Human Services, Public Health Service, 1991; DHHS Publication No. (PHS) 91-50212.

Department of Health and Social Security. *Sharing resources for health in England: report of the Resource Allocation Working Party.* London: HMSO, 1976.

Department of Health, Education, and Welfare. *Healthy People: The Surgeon-General's Report on Health Promotion and Disease Prevention.* Washington, DC: Department of Health, Education, and Welfare, 1979; Publication No. (PHS) 79-55071.

Desenclos DJ, Hubert B. Limitations to the universal use of capture–recapture methods. *Int J Epidemiol* 1994;23:1322–3.

Detels R, Holland WW, McEwen J, Omenn GS (eds). *Oxford Textbook of Public Health,* 3rd ed. New York: Oxford University Press, 1997.

Diehr P, Cain K, Ye Z, Abdul-Salam F. Small-area variation statistics: methods for comparing several DRGs. *Med Care* 1993;31 (Suppl):YS45–YS53.

Dietz-Rioux A, Benach J, Tapia JA. Should policy recommendations be excluded from epidemiologic research papers [letter]? *Epidemiology* 1994;5: 637–8.

Donabedian A. *The Definition of Quality and Approaches to its Assessment.* Ann Arbor, MI: Health Administration Press, 1980.

Drummond MF, Stoddart GL, Torrance GW. *Methods for the Economic Evaluation of Health Care Programmes.* Oxford: Oxford Medical Publications, 1987.

Dubos R. *Man Adapting.* New Haven: Yale University Press, 1965.

Dunn WN. *Public Policy. An Introduction.* Englewood Cliffs, NJ: Prentice-Hall, 1981.

Eddy DM. Setting priorities for cancer control programs. *J Natl Cancer Inst* 1986;76:187–99.

Eddy DM. Oregon's methods: did cost-effectiveness analysis fail? *JAMA* 1991;266:2135–41.

Egger M, Schneider M, Davey Smith G. Spurious precision? Meta-analysis of observational studies. *BMJ* 1998;316:140–4.

Estève J, Benhamou E, Raymond L. *Statistical Methods in Cancer Research, Vol. IV. Descriptive Epidemiology. IARC Sci Publ* 1994;128.

Etzioni A. Mixed-scanning: a "third" approach to decision making. *Public Admin Rev* 1967;27:385–92.

EuroQol Group. EuroQol—a new facility for the measurement of health-related quality of life. *Health Policy* 1990;16:199–208.

Evans RG, Barer ML, Marmor TR (eds). *Why Are Some People Healthy and Others Not? The Determinants of Health of Populations.* New York: Aldine de Gruyter, 1994.

Evans RG, Stoddart GL. Producing health, consuming health care. In Evans RG, Barer ML, Marmor TR. *Why Are Some People Healthy and Others Not? The Determinants of Health of Populations.* New York: Aldine de Gruyter, 1994;27–64.

Eyles J, Birch S. A population needs-based approach to health-care resource allocation and planning in Ontario: a link between policy goals and practice? *Can J Public Health* 1993;84:112-7.

Eyles J, Birch S, Chambers S, Hurley J, Hutchison B. A needs-based methodology for allocating health care resources in Ontario, Canada: development and an application. *Soc Sci Med* 1991;33:489–500.

Flanders D. Basic (statistical) models of disease occurrence. *Int J Epidemiol* 1995;24:1–7.

Foot D. *Boom, Bust & Echo: How to Profit from the Coming Demographic Shift.* Toronto: Macfarlane Walter & Ross, 1996.

Frankish CJ, Green LW, Ratner PA, Chomik T, Larsen C. *Health Impact Assessment as a Tool for Population Health Promotion and Public Policy.* A Report submitted to the Health Promotion Development Division of Health Canada. Vancouver: Institute of Health Promotion Research, University of British Columbia, May 1996.

Friede A, Blum HL, McDonald M. Public health informatics: how information-age technology can strengthen public health. *Annu Rev Public Health* 1995;16:239–52.

Fries JF. Aging, natural death, and the compression of morbidity. *N Engl J Med* 1980;303:130–35.

Gafni A, Birch S. Guidelines for the adoption of new technologies: a prescription for uncontrolled growth in expenditures and how to avoid the problem. *Can Med Assoc J* 1993;148:913–7.

Goel V, Williams JI, Anderson GM, Blackstien-Hirsch P, Fooks C, Naylor CD. *Patterns of Health Care in Ontario: The ICES Practice Atlas,* 2nd ed. Toronto: Institute for Clinical Evaluative Sciences, 1996.

Goodman C. It's time to rethink health care technology assessment. *Int J Technol Assess Health Care* 1992;8:335–58.

Goodman SN. Meta-analysis in health services research. In: Armenian HK, Shapiro S (eds). *Epidemiology and Health Services.* New York: Oxford University Press, 1998;229–59.

Government Committee on Choices in Health Care. *Choices in Health Care. A Report by the Government Committee on Choices in Health Care.* Rijswijk, The Netherlands: Ministry of Welfare, Health and Cultural Affairs, 1992.

Greenland S. Some popular meta-analytic methods. *Am J Epidemiol* 1994; 290–6.

Gregg MB, Dicker RC, Goodman RA (eds). *Field Epidemiology.* New York: Oxford University Press, 1996.

Gunning-Schepers L. The health benefits of prevention: a simulation approach. *Health Policy* 1989:12:1–221.

Gunning-Schepers LJ. Notes from course in Epidemiology and Health Policy, Erasmus Summer Programme, Erasmus University, Rotterdam, 1995:24.

Guyatt GH, Sackett DL, Cook DJ, for the Evidence-Based Medicine Working Group. Users' guides to the medical literature. II. How to use an article about therapy or prevention. A. are the results valid? *JAMA* 1993;270: 2598–601.

Guyatt GH, Sackett DL, Cook DJ, for the Evidence-Based Medicine Working Group. Users' guides to the medical literature. II. How to use an article about therapy or prevention: B. What were the results and will they help me in caring for my patients? *JAMA* 1994;271;59–63.

Guyatt GH, Sackett DL, Sinclair JC, Hayward R, Cook DJ, Cook RJ, for the Evidence-Based Working Group. Users' guides to the medical literature. IX. A method of grading health care recommendations. *JAMA* 1995;274:1800–4.

Gyorkos TW, Tannenbaum TN, Abrahamowicz M, Oxman AD, Scott EAF, et al. An approach to the development of practice guidelines for community health interventions. *Can J Public Health* 1994; 85 (Suppl 1):S8–S13.

Haber M, Watelet L, Halloran ME. On individual and population effectiveness of vaccination. *Int J Epidemiol* 1995;24:1249–60.

Hadorn DC, Baker D, Hodges JS, Hicks N. Rating the quality of evidence for clinical practice guidelines. *J Clin Epidemiol* 1996;49:749–54.

Halperin W, Baker EL Jr. *Public Health Surveillance*. New York: van Nostrand Reinhold, 1992.

Hanlon J. Pickett G. *Public Health Administration and Practice*. Santa Clara, CA: Times Mirror/Mosby College Publishing, 1984.

Hayes MV, Dunn JR. *Population Health In Canada: A Systematic Review*. Ottawa: Canadian Policy Research Networks Study No. H I 01 I, 1998.

Health and Welfare Canada, Statistics Canada. *Mortality Atlas of Canada, Vol. 3: Urban Mortality*. Ottawa: Supply and Services Canada, 1984.

Health for All Australians: Report of the Health Targets and Implementation (Health for All) Committee to Australian Health Ministers. Canberra: Australian Government Publishing Service, 1988.

Health Services Restructuring Commission. *Ottawa Health Services Restructuring Report*. Toronto: Health Services Restructuring Commission, February 1997.

Helfenstein U. The use of transfer function models, intervention analysis and related time series methods in epidemiology. *Int J Epidemiol* 1991; 20:808–15.

Herbert ME. *Modelling Future Mortality in Ontario: Extension of the PREVENT Model and development of an Ontario database*. University of Ottawa MSc thesis, Department of Epidemiology and Community Medicine, 1994.

Hertz-Picciotto I. Epidemiology and quantitative risk assessment: a bridge from science to policy. *Am J Public Health* 1995;85:484–91.

Hill GB. Computer monitoring of cancer incidence. *Chron Dis Can* 1983;4: 40–2.

Holford TR. Understanding the effects of age, period, and cohort on incidence and mortality rates. *Annu Rev Public Health* 1991;12:425–57.

Holland WW, Wainwright AH. Epidemiology and health policy. *Epidemiol Rev* 1979;1:211–32.

Hook EB, Regal RR. The value of capture-recapture methods even for apparent exhaustive surveys: the need for adjustment for source of ascertainment intersection in attempted complete prevalence studies. *Am J Epidemiol* 1992;135:1060–7.

Hox JJ. *Applied Multilevel Analysis*. Amsterdam: TT-Publikaties, 1995.

Hunink MGM, Goldman L, Tosteson ANA, Mittleman MA, Goldman PA, Williams LW, Tsevat J, Weinstein MC. The recent decline in mortality from coronary heart disease, 1980–1990: the effect of secular trends in risk factors and treatment. *JAMA* 1997;277:535–42.

Ibrahim, MA. *Epidemiology and Health Policy*. Rockville, MD: Aspen Systems Corporation, 1985.

Idler EL, Benyamini Y. Self-rated health and mortality: a review of twenty-seven community studies. *J Health Soc Behav* 1997;38:21–37.

International Working Group for Disease Monitoring and Forecasting. Capture-recapture and multiple-record systems estimation. I. History and theoretical development. II. Applications in human diseases. *Am J Epidemiol* 1995; 142:1047–68.

Jordan J, Dowsell T, Harrison S, Lilford RJ, Mort M. Whose priorities? Listening to users and the public. *BMJ* 1998; 316: 1668–70.

Kennedy BP, Kawachi I, Prothrow-Smith D. Income distribution and mortality: cross sectional ecological study of the Robin Hood Index in the United States. *BMJ* 1996;312:1004–29.

Kilpatrick SJ. The distribution of episodes of illness—a research tool in general practice? *J R Coll Gen Practitioners* 1975;25:686–90.

Kitzhaber JA. Prioritising health services in an era of limits: the Oregon experience. *BMJ* 1993;307:373–7.

Kleinbaum DG, Kupper LL, Morgenstern H. *Epidemiologic Research: Principles and Quantitative Methods*. Belmont, CA: Lifetime Learning Publications, 1982.

Korn EL, Graubard BI. Epidemiologic studies utilizing surveys: accounting for the sampling design. *Am J Public Health* 1991;81:1166–73.

Krieger N. The making of public health data: paradigms, politics, and policy. *J Public Health Policy* 1992;13: 412–27.

Kuller LH. Epidemiology and health policy. *Am J Epidemiol* 1988;127:2–16.

Kuller L. The use of existing databases in morbidity and mortality studies [editorial]. *Am J Public Health* 1995;85:1198–1200.

Kupper LL, Janis JM, Karmous A, Greenberg BG. Statistical age-period-cohort analysis: a review and critique. *J Chron Dis* 1985;38:811–30.

Lalonde M. *A New Perspective on the Health of Canadians*. Ottawa: Information Canada, 1974.

Lamberts H, Wood M (eds). *International Classification of Primary Care*. Oxford: Oxford University Press, 1987.

Laporte RE, Tull ES, McCarty D. Monitoring the incidence of myocardial infarctions: application of capture-mark-recapture technology. *Int J Epidemiol* 1992;21: 258–63.

Laporte RE. Global public health and the information superhighway. *BMJ* 1994;308:1651–2.

Last JM. New pathways in an age of ecological and ethical concerns. *Int J Epidemiol* 1994;23:1–4.

Last JM (ed). *A Dictionary of Epidemiology*, 3rd ed. New York: Oxford University Press, 1995.

Last JM, Wallace R (eds). *Maxcy-Rosenau-Last Public Health and Preventive Medicine*, 13th ed. Norwalk, CT: Appleton & Lange, 1992.

Lau J, Schmid CH, Chalmers TC. Cumulative meta-analysis of clinical trials builds evidence for exemplary medical care. *J Clin Epidemiol* 1995;48: 45–57.

Laupacis A, Feeny D, Detsky AS, Tugwell PX. How attractive does a new technology have to be to warrant adoption and utilization? Tentative guidelines for using clinical and economic evaluations. *Can Med Assoc J* 1992;146:473–81.

Laupacis A, Feeny D, Detsky AS, Tugwell PX. Tentative guidelines for using clinical and economic evaluations revisited. *Can Med Assoc J* 1993;148:927–9.

Laupacis A, Sackett DL, Roberts RS. An assessment of clinically useful measures of the consequences of treatment. *N Engl J Med* 1988; 318:1728–33.

Leavell HR, Clark EG. *Preventive Medicine for the Doctor in His Community: An Epidemiologic Approach*. New York: McGraw-Hill, 1965.

Leeder SR. The contribution of epidemiology to the definition of health goals and targets for Australia. *Int J Epidemiol* 1995;24 (Suppl 1):S109–S112.

Levine M, Walter S, Lee H, Haines T, Holbrook A, Moyer V. Users' Guides to the medical literature. IV. How to use an article about harm. *JAMA* 1994;271;1615–9.

Levine S, Lilienfeld A. Introduction. In: Levine S, Lilienfeld A (eds). *Epidemiology and Health Policy*. New York and London: Tavistock, 1987:1–14.

Lindblom CE. The science of muddling through. *Public Admin Rev* 1959;19: 79–88.

Lindblom CE. Still muddling, not yet through. *Public Admin Rev* 1979;39: 517–26.

Lindblom CE. *The policy-making process*, 2nd ed. Englewood Cliffs, NJ: Prentice-Hall, 1980.

Lohr KN. Outcome measurement: concepts and questions. *Inquiry* 1988;25: 37–50.

Lomas J. Reticent rationers: consumer input to health care priorities. In: Gunning-Schepers LJ, Kronjee GJ, Spasoff RA (eds). *Fundamental Questions about the Future of Health Care*. The Hague: Netherlands Scientific Council for Government Policy, 1996:71–85.

Lucaciu D. *Overview of the Taxation Family File (T1FF) Processing*. Statistics Canada, Small Area and Administrative Data Division, April 1993.

Lynge E. New draft on European Directive on confidential data. *BMJ* 1995;310:1024.

Mackenbach JP, Kunst AE. Measuring the magnitude of socio-economic inequalities in health: an overview of available measures illustrated with two examples from Europe. *Soc Sci Med* 1997;44:757–71.

Mackenzie EA, Shapiro S, Yaffe R. The utility of synthetic and regression estimation. Techniques for local health planning. *Med Care* 1985;23:1–13.

Mao Y, McCourt C, Morrison H, Pepin-Laplante O, Semenciw R, Silins J, Spasoff RA, Trempe N, Wigle D. Community-based mortality surveillance: the Maniwaki experience. Investigation of excess mortality in a community. *Can J Public Health* 1984:75:429–33.

Marmor TR, Boyum D. Medical care and public policy: the benefits and burdens of asking fundamental questions. In: Gunning-Schepers LJ, Kronjee GJ, Spasoff RA (eds). *Fundamental Questions about the Future of Health Care*. The Hague: Netherlands Scientific Council for Government Policy 1996:89–104.

Marmot MG, Davey Smith G. Why are the Japanese living longer? *BMJ* 1989;299:1547–51.

Marmot MG, Shipley MJ, Rose G. Inequalities in death—specific explanations of a general pattern? *Lancet* 1984;1:1003–6.

Maslow AH. *Toward a Psychology of Being,* 2nd ed. New York: van Nostrand Reinhold, 1968.

Mayer RR, Greenwood E. *The Design of Social Policy Research.* Englewood Cliffs, NJ: Prentice-Hall, 1980.

Maynard A. Evidence-based medicine: an incomplete method for informing treatment choices. *Lancet* 1997;349:126–8.

McDowell IW, Newell C. *Measuring Health: A Guide to Rating Scales and Questionnaires,* 2nd ed. New York: Oxford University Press, 1996.

McGinnis JM, Harrell JA, Artz LM, Files AA, Maiese DR. Objectives-based strategies for disease prevention. In: Detels R, Holland WW, McEwen J, Omenn GS (eds). *Oxford Textbook of Public Health, 3rd ed,* Vol. 3. New York: Oxford University Press, 1997:1621–31.

McGlynn EA, Kosecoff J, Brook RH. Format and conduct of consensus development conferences. *Int J Technol Assess Health Care* 1990;6:450–69.

McLean M, Duclos P, Jacob P, Humphreys P. Incidence of Guillain-Barre syndrome in Ontario and Quebec, 1983–1989, using hospital service databases. *Epidemiology* 1994;5:443–8.

McPherson K, Wennberg J, Hovind O, Clifford P. Small-area variations in the use of common surgical procedures: an international comparison of New England, England, and Norway. *N Engl J Med* 1982;307:1310–4.

Mehrez A, Gafni A. Quality adjusted life years, utility theory, and healthy years equivalents. *Med decis Making* 1989;9:142–9.

Miettinen OS. Proportion of disease caused or prevented by a given exposure trait or intervention. *Am J Epidemiol* 1974;99:325–32.

Millar WJ, David P. *Life Tables, Canada and the Provinces, 1990–92.* Statistics Canada Occasional Publication 84-537. Ottawa: Minister of Industry, 1995.

Ministry of Treasury and Economics. *Demographic Bulletin: Population Projections for Regional Municipalities, Counties and Districts of Ontario to 2011.* Toronto: Ministry of Treasury and Economics, 1989.

Moody PE. *Decision Making: Proven Methods for Better Decisions.* New York: McGraw-Hill, 1983.

Moore R, Mao Y, Zhang J, Clarke K. *Economic Burden of Illness in Canada, 1993.* Ottawa: Canadian Public Health Association, 1997.

Morgenstern H. Uses of ecologic analysis in epidemiologic research. *Am J Public Health* 1982;72:1136–1344.

Morgenstern H. Ecologic studies in epidemiology: concepts, principles, and methods. *Annu Rev Public Health* 1995;16:61–81.

Morrison AS. *Screening in Chronic Disease,* 2nd ed. New York: Oxford University Press, 1992.

Morse JM, Field PA. *Qualitative Research Methods for Health Professionals,* 2nd ed. Thousand Oaks, CA: Sage Publications, 1995.

Moser C, Kalton G. *Survey Methods in Social Investigation.* London: Heinemann Educational Books, 1971.

Mosteller F, Colditz GA. Understanding research synthesis (meta-analysis). *Annu Rev Public Health* 1996;17:1–23.

Muir Gray JAM. *Evidence-based Healthcare: How to make health policy and management decisions.* New York: Churchill Livingstone, 1997.

Murnaghan JH. Health indicators and information systems for the year 2000. *Annu Rev Public Health* 1981;2:299–361.

Murray CJL. Quantifying the burden of disease: the technical basis for disability-adjusted life years. *Bull World Health Organ* 1994;72:429–445.

Murray CJL, Lopez AD. Quantifying disability: data, methods and results. *Bull World Health Organ* 1994;72:481–94.

Murray CJL, Lopez AD. Evidence-based health policy—lessons from the Global Burden of Disease study. *Science* 1996a;274:740–3.

Murray CJL, Lopez AD (eds). *The Global Burden of Disease, Vol. I. A Comprehensive Assessment of Mortality and Disability from Diseases, Injuries and Risk Factors, in 1990 and Projected to 2020.* Cambridge, MA: Harvard University Press, 1996b.

National Institute of Epidemiology. *Public Health Common Data Set 1996, England*, Vol. I. London: Department of Health, 1997.

National Research Council, Committee on the Institutional Means for Assessment of Risks to Public Health. *Risk Assessment in the Federal Government: Managing the Process.* Washington, DC: National Academy Press, 1983.

National Task Force on Health Information. *Report of the Project Team on Health Information Analysis: Potentials and Impediments.* Ottawa: Statistics Canada, 6 September 1991.

National Task Force on Health Information. *Report of the Project Team on Information Required to Understand the Determinants of Health.* Ottawa: Statistics Canada, 21 April 1992.

Naylor CD, Williams JI, Basinski A, Goel V. Technology assessment and cost-effectiveness: misguided guidelines? *Can Med Assoc J* 1993;148:921–4.

Needs/Impact-Based Planning Committee. *A Guide to Needs/Impact-Based Planning.* Toronto: Ontario Ministry of Health, Community Health Division, 1996.

Neufeld VR, Spasoff RA. The role and function of Health Intelligence Units. In: White KL, Connelly JE (eds). *The Medical School's Mission and the Population's Health. Medical Education in Canada, the United Kingdom, the United States, and Australia.* New York: Springer-Verlag, 1992:113–31.

Newcombe H. *Handbook of Record Linkage: Methods for Health and Statistical Studies, Administration, and Business.* New York: Oxford Medical Publications, 1988.

Newcombe HB. When "privacy" threatens public health. *Can J Public Health* 1995;86:188–92.

Nova Scotia–Saskatchewan Cardiovascular Disease Epidemiology Group. Estimation of the incidence of acute myocardial infarction using record linkage: a feasibility study in Nova Scotia and Saskatchewan. *Can J Public Health* 1989;80:412–7.

Nusselder WJ, van der Velden K, van Sonsbeek JL, Lenior ME, van den Bos GAM. The elimination of selected chronic diseases in a population: the compression and expansion of morbidity. *Am J Public Health* 1996;86(2): 187–94.

O'Campo P, Xue X, Wang M-C, Caughy MO. Neighborhood risk factors for low birthweight in Baltimore: a multilevel analysis. *Am J Public Health* 1997;87:1113–8.

Office of Disease Prevention and Health Promotion. *The 1990 Health Objectives for the Nation: A Midcourse Review.* Washington, DC: Department of Health and Human Services, Public Health Service, 1986.

Olsen J, on behalf of the International Epidemiology Association. Directive of the European Parliament and of the Council on the Protection of Individuals with Regard to the Processing of Personal Data and on the Free Movement of Such Data [letter]. *Int J Epidemiol* 1995;24:462–3.

Omenn G. The role of environmental epidemiology in public policy. *Ann Epidemiol* 1993;3:319–22.

Oortmarssen GJ van, Habbema JDF, van der Maas PJ, de Koning HJ, Collette HJA, Verbeek ALM, Geerts AT, Lubbe KTN. A model for breast cancer screening. *Cancer* 1990;66:1601–12.

Oxman AD, Cook DJ, Guyatt GH, for the Evidence-Based Medicine Working Group. Users' guides to the medical literature. VI. How to use an overview. *JAMA* 1994;272;1367–71.

Oxman AD, Sackett DL, Guyatt GH for the Evidence-Based Medicine Working Group. Users' guides to the medical literature. I. How to get started. *JAMA* 1993;270:2093–5.

Pal LA. *Public Policy Analysis.* 2nd ed. Scarborough: Nelson Canada, 1992.

Papoz L, Balkau B, Lellouch J. Case counting in epidemiology: limitations of methods based on multiple data sources. *Int J Epidemiol* 1996;25:474–8.

Patrick DL, Bergner M. Measurement of health status in the 1990s. *Annu Rev Public Health* 1990;11:165–83.

Patrick DL, Erickson P. *Health Status and Health Policy: Quality of Life in Health Care Evaluation and Resource Allocation.* New York: Oxford University Press, 1993.

Pearce N. What does the odds ratio estimate in a case–control study? *Int J Epidemiol* 1993;22:1189–92.

Penchansky R, Thomas JW. The concept of access: definition and relationship to consumer satisfaction. *Med Care* 1981;19:127–40.

Peron Y, Strohmenger C. *Demographic and Health Indicators: Presentation and Interpretation.* Ottawa: Statistics Canada, 1985 (Catalogue No. 82-543E).

Peto R, Collins R, Gray R. Large-scale randomized evidence: large, simple trials and overviews of trials. *J Clin Epidemiol* 1995;48:23–40.

Petitti DB. *Meta-analysis, Decision Analysis, and Cost-Effectiveness Analysis: Methods for Quantitative Synthesis in Medicine.* New York: Oxford University Press, 1994.

Pickin C, St Leger S. *Assessing Health Using the Life Cycle Framework.* Buckingham and Philadelphia: Open University Press, 1993.

Porteous NL, Sheldrick BJ, Stewart PJ. *Program Evaluation Tool Kit: A Blueprint for Public Health Management.* Ottawa: Ottawa-Carleton Health Department, 1997.

Premier's Council on Health Strategy. *A Vision of Health: Health Goals for Ontario.* Toronto: Premier's Council on Health Strategy, 1990.

Purcell NJ, Kish L. Estimation for small domains. *Biometrics* 1979;35:365–84.

Remington PL. Communicating epidemiologic information. In: Brownson RC, Petitti DB (eds). *Applied Epidemiology: Theory to Practice.* New York: Oxford University Press, 1998:323–48.

Rice DP. *Estimating the Cost of Illness.* Health Economics Series #6. Washington, DC: Department of Health Education and Welfare, 1966.

Richmond JB, Kotelchuck M. Coordination and development of strategies and policy for health promotion in the United States. In: Holland WW, Detels R, Knox G (eds). *Oxford Textbook of Public Health,* Vol. I, 2nd ed. New York: Oxford University Press, 1991:441–54.

Roemer MI. Bed supply and hospital utilization: a natural experiment. *Hospitals* 1961;35:36–42.

Rogan WJ, Gladen B. Estimating prevalence from the results of a screening test. *Am J Epidemiol* 1978;107:71–6.

Roos NP. Linking patients to hospitals. Defining urban hospital service populations. *Med Care* 1993:31(5; Suppl):YS6–YS15.

Roos NP, Black CD, Frohlich N, Decoster C, Cohen MM, Tataryn DJ, Mustard CA, Toll F, Carriere KC, Burchill CA, MacWilliam MSc, Bogdanovic B. A population-based health information system. *Med Care* 1995;33(12, Suppl): DS13–DS20.

Roos NP, Roos LL. High and low surgical rates: risk factors for area residents. *Am J Public Health* 1981;71:591–600.

Roos NP, Shapiro E (eds.) Health and health care: experience with a population-based health information system. *Med Care* 1995;33(12, Suppl): DS1–DS146.

Rose G. Sick individuals and sick populations. *Int J Epidemiol* 1985;14:32–8.

Rose G. *The Strategy of Preventive Medicine.* Oxford: Oxford University Press, 1992.

Rosén M. *Epidemiology in Planning for Health.* Stockholm: Swedish Planning and Rationalization Institute for Health and Social Services, 1987.

Rosén M, Nystrom L, Wall S. Guidelines for regional mortality analysis: an epidemiological approach to health planning. *Int J Epidemiol* 1985;14(2): 293–9.

Rothman KJ. Policy recommendations in research papers [editorial]. *Epidemiology* 1993;4:94–5.

Rothman KJ, Poole C. Science and policy making [editorial]. *Am J Public Health* 1985;75:340–1.

Rowan K. Global questions and scores. In: Jenkinson C (ed). *Measuring Health and Medical Outcomes.* London: UCL Press, 1994;54–67.

Russell LB. *Is Prevention Better than Cure?* Washington, DC: Brookings Institution, 1986.

Rutstein DD, Berenberg W, Chalmers TC, Child CG, Fishman AP, Perrin EB. Measuring the quality of medical care. A clinical method. *N Engl J Med* 1976;294:582–8.

Ruwaard D, Kramers PGN, van den Berg Jeths A, Achterberg PW. *Public*

Health Status and Forecasts. The Health status of the Dutch population over the period 1950–2010. Bilthoven, The Netherlands: National Institute of Public Health and Environmental Protection, 1994.

Sackett DL, Haynes RB, Guyatt GH, Tugwell P. *Clinical Epidemiology. A Basic Science for Clinical Medicine,* 2nd ed. Boston: Little Brown, 1991.

Sackett DL, Richardson WS, Rosenberg W, Haynes RB. *Evidence-based Medicine: How to Practise and Teach EBM.* New York: Churchill Livingstone, 1997.

Sainfort F, Remington PL. The disease impact assessment system (DIAS). *Public Health Rep* 1995;110:639–44.

Samet JM, Burke TA. Epidemiology and risk assessment. In: Brownson RC, Petitti DB (eds). *Applied Epidemiology: Theory to Practice.* New York: Oxford University Press, 1998:137–75.

Scholten HJ, de Lepper MJC. The benefits of the application of geographical information systems in public and environmental health. *World Health Stat Q* 1991;44:160–9.

Schwartz S. The fallacy of the ecologic fallacy: the potential misuse of a concept and the consequences. *Am J Public Health* 1994;84:819–824.

Selvin S. *Statistical Analysis of Epidemiologic Data.* New York: Oxford University Press, 1991.

Shapiro S. Epidemiology and public policy. *Am J Epidemiol* 1991;134:1057–61.

Shapiro S. Meta-analysis/shmeta-analysis. *Am J Epidemiol* 1994;140:771–8. [Also see related comments, pp 779–91.]

Shortell SM, Solomon MA. Improving health care policy research. *J Health Politics, Policy Law* 1982;6:684–702.

Shyrock HS, Siegel JS and associates. *The Methods and Materials of Demography* (condensed edition by Stockwell EG). New York: Academic Press, 1976.

Smith G. Development of rapid epidemiologic assessment methods to evaluate health status and delivery of health services. *Int J Epidemiol* 1989; 18: (Suppl 2):S2–S15.

Spasoff RA, Gilkes DT. Up-to-date denominators: evaluation of Taxation Family File for public health planning. *Can J Public Health* 1994;85:413–7.

Spasoff RA, McDowell IW. Estimating the combined effect of several disease precursors in Health Risk Appraisal. *Am J Prevent Med* 1987;3:182–9.

Spasoff RA, Strike C, Dunkley GC, Nair, Boulet JR. Small group estimation for public health. *Can J Public Health* 1996;87:130–4.

Spitzer WO, Letouzé D, Spasoff RA, Williams JI. Evaluating new methods for provision of primary care: an Ontario strategy. *Med Care* 1978;16:560–73.

Stallones RA. To advance epidemiology. *Annu Rev Public Health* 1980;1:69–82.

Statistics Canada. *Population Projections for Canada, Provinces and Territories, 1989–2011.* Ottawa: Supply and Services Canada, 1990 (Statistics Canada Catalogue #91-520).

Statistics Canada. *1991 Census Catalogue.* Ottawa: Statistics Canada, 1992 (Catalogue #92-302E).

Stephens T, Fowler Graham D (eds). *Canada's Health Promotion Survey 1990: Technical Report.* Ottawa: Minister of Supply and Services Canada, 1993.

Stevens A, Raftery J. *Health Care Needs Assessment: The Epidemiologically Based*

Needs Assessment Reviews, Vol. 1. Oxford and New York: Radcliffe Medical Press, 1994.

Stroup D. Special analytic issues. In: Teutsch SM, Churchill RE. *Principles and Practice of Health Surveillance.* New York: Oxford University Press, 1994: 136–49.

Stroup DF, Thacker SB. A Bayesian approach to the detection of aberrations in public health surveillance data. *Epidemiology* 1993;4:435–43.

Sullivan DF. A single index of mortality and morbidity. *HSMHA Health Rep* 1971;86:347– 54.

Susser M. The logical in ecological. I. The logic of analysis. II. The logic of design. *Am J Public Health* 1994;84:819–24.

Swift M, Nishri D. Using SAS/GRAPH software to create unclassed choropleth maps. Ontario Cancer Treatment and Research Foundation. Presented at the SAS Users Group International 18th annual conference, May 9–12, 1993, New York, NY.

Syme L, Guralik JL. Epidemiology and health policy: coronary heart disease. In: Levine S, Lilienfeld A (eds). *Epidemiology and Health Policy.* New York and London: Tavistock, 1987:85–116.

Symposium on Community Intervention Trials. *Am J Epidemiol* 1995;142: 567–99.

Task Force on the Allocation of Health Care Resources. *Investigation of the Impact of Demographic Change on the Health Care System in Canada. Final Report.* Ottawa: Canadian Medical Association, August 1984.

Taubes G. Epidemiology faces its limits. *Science* 1995;269:164–9.

Teret S. So what? [editorial]. *Epidemiology* 1993;4:93–4.

Terris M. Epidemiology as a guide to health policy. *Annu Rev Public Health* 1980;1:323–44.

Teutsch SM, Churchill RE. *Principles and Practice of Public Health Surveillance.* New York: Oxford University Press, 1994.

Toronto Working Group on Cholesterol Policy, for the Task Force on the Use and Provision of Medical Services. *Detection and Management of Asymptomatic Hypercholesterolemia.* Toronto: Ontario Ministry of Health and Ontario Medical Association, 1989.

Torrance GW. The measurement of health state utilities for economic appraisal: a review. *J Health Econ* 1986;5:1–30.

Townsend P, Davidson N (eds). *The Black Report.* Reprinted in *Inequalities in Health.* Harmondsworth: Penguin Books, 1992.

Trochim WMK. The regression-discontinuity design. In: Sechrest L, Perrin E, Bunker J (eds). *Research Methodology: Strengthening Causal Interpretations of Nonexperimental Data* (Conference Proceedings). Washington, DC: U.S. Department of Health and Human Services, Public Health Service, 1990:119–39.

Tugwell P, Bennett KJ, Sackett DL, Haynes RB. The Measurement Iterative Loop: a framework for the critical appraisal of need, benefits and costs of health interventions. *J Chron Dis* 1985;38:339–51.

United Nations. *Age and sex patterns of mortality: model life tables for underdeveloped countries.* Population Studies, Series A, No. 22, 1955.

U.S. Congress. Office of Technology Assessment. *Strategies for medical technology assessment.* Washington, DC: U.S. Government Printing Office, 1982.

U.S. Preventive Services Task Force. *Guide to Clinical Preventive Services,* 2nd ed. Baltimore: Williams & Wilkins, 1996.

van der Grinten TED. Scope for policy: essence, operation and reform of the policy system of Dutch health care. In: Gunning-Schepers LJ, Kronjee GJ, Spasoff RA (eds). *Fundamental Questions about the Future of Health Care.* The Hague: Netherlands Scientific Council for Government Policy, 1996;135–54.

van der Maas P, Hofman A, Dekker E (eds). *Epidemiologie en Gezondheidsbeleid* (Epidemiology and Health Policy). Alphen aan de Rijn: Samson Stafleu, 1989.

van de Mheen PJ, Gunning-Schepers LJ. Differences between studies in reported relative risks associated with smoking: an overview. *Public Health Rep* 1996;111:420–6.

van de Mheen PJ, Gunning-Schepers LJ. Assuming independence of risk factor prevalences in simulation models like PREVENT: when are the outcomes seriously biased? *Eur J Public Health* 1997;7:216–220.

van Wyck P, Hockin JC. Mortality surveillance: an integral part of quality assurance. *Health Manage Forum* 1984;5:27–36.

Vickers G. What sets the goals of public health? *Lancet* 1958;1:599–604.

Wagstaff A, Paci P, van Doorslaer E. On the measurement of inequalities in health. *Soc Sci Med* 1991;33:545–57.

Walt G. *Health Policy: An Introduction to Process and Power.* London and New Jersey: Zed Books, 1994.

Walter SD. Effects of interaction, confounding and observation error on attributable risk estimation. *Am J Epidemiol* 1983;117:598–604.

Walter SD, Birnie SE. Mapping mortality and morbidity patterns: an international comparison. *Int J Epidemiol* 1991;20:678–89.

Ware JE, Sherbourne CD. The MOS 36-item Short-Form Health Survey (SF-36). I. Conceptual framework and item selection. *Med Care* 1992;30:473–83.

Weed DL. Science, ethics guidelines and advocacy in epidemiology. *Ann Epidemiol* 1994;4:166–71.

Weinstein MC, Coxson PG, Williams LW, Pass TM, Stason WB, Goldman L. Forecasting coronary heart disease incidence, mortality, and cost: the Coronary Heart Disease Policy Model. *Am J Public Health* 1987;77:1417–26.

Wennberg J, Gittelsohn A. Variations in medical care among small areas. *Sci Am* 1982;246:120–34.

Wilkin D, Hallam I, Daggett M. *Measures of Need and Outcome for Primary Health Care.* Oxford: Oxford University Press, 1992.

Wilkins R, Adams O. *Healthfulness of Life.* Montreal: Institute for Research on Public Policy, 1983.

Willett W. *Nutritional Epidemiology,* 2nd ed. New York: Oxford University Press, 1998.

Williams JI, Young W. A summary of studies on the quality of health care administrative databases in Canada. In: Goel V, Williams JI, Anderson GM, Blackstein-Hirsch P, Fooks C, Naylor CD. *Patterns of Health Care in Ontario: The ICES Practice Atlas*, 2nd ed. Toronto: Institute for Clinical Evaluative Sciences, 1996:339–45.

Wilson JMG, Jungner G. *The Principles and Practice of Screening for Disease.* Geneva: World Health Organization Public Health Papers #34, 1968.

Winkelstein W, Marmot M. Primary prevention of ischemic heart disease: evaluation of community interventions. *Annu Rev Public Health* 1981;2: 253–76.

Wolfson MC. A template for health information. *World Health Stat Q* 1992;45: 109–113.

Wolfson M. POHEM—a framework for modeling and understanding the health of human populations. *World Health Stat Q* 1994;47:157–76.

Working Group on Community Health Information Systems. *Health Status Indicators: Definitions and Interpretations.* Ottawa: Canadian Institute for Health Information, 1995.

Working Group on the Prevention and Control of Cardiovascular Disease. *Promoting Heart Health in Canada: A Focus on Cholesterol.* Ottawa: Health Canada, November 1992.

World Health Organization. The Constitution of the World Health Organization. *WHO Chron* 1947;1:29.

World Health Organization. *International Classification of Impairments, Disabilities and Handicaps. A Manual of Classification Relating to the Consequences of Disease.* Geneva: World Health Organization, 1980.

World Health Organization. *Global Strategy for Health for All by the Year 2000.* Geneva: World Health Organization, Health for All Series No. 3, 1981a.

World Health Organization. *Health Programme Evaluation: Guiding Principles for its Application in the Managerial Process for National Health Development.* Geneva: World Health Organization, Health for All Series No. 6, 1981b.

World Health Organization. *Targets for Health for All 2000.* Copenhagen: World Health Organization Regional Office for Europe, 1985.

World Health Organization. *Ottawa Charter for Health Promotion.* Ottawa: World Health Organization, Health and Welfare Canada and Canadian Public Health Association, 1986.

World Health Organization. *International Statistical Classification of Diseases and Related Health Problems*, 10th rev. Geneva: World Health Organization, 1992.

World Health Organization. *Terminology for the European Health Policy Conference. A glossary with equivalents in French, German and Russian.* Copenhagen: World Health Organization Regional Office for Europe, 1994 (ICP/HSC 419).

Wright J, Williams R, Wilkinson JR. Development and importance of health needs assessment. *BMJ* 1998;316:1310–3.

Wynder EL. Invited commentary: Response to *Science* article "Epidemiology faces its limits". *Am J Epidemiol* 1996;143:747–9.

Index